Learning from
Paediatric
Patient Journeys

Pediatric Diagnosis and Management
Series Editors: James F. Bale Jr. and Stephen D. Marks

NEW AND FORTHCOMING TITLES

Learning from
Paediatric
Patient Journeys

What children and their families can tell us

Edited by

Dr Chloe Macaulay, BA, MBBS, MRCPCH, MSc, PGCertMedEd
Consultant Paediatrician, Evelina Children's Hospital, London, UK
and
Former teaching fellow UCL iBSc in
Paediatrics and Child Health, London (2010-2012)

Dr Polly Powell, MBChB, MRCPCH, PGCertMedEd
Paediatric Trainee, London, UK
and
Former teaching fellow UCL iBSc in
Paediatrics and Child Health, London (2012-2013)

Dr Caroline Fertleman, BA, MB BChir, MSc, FRCPCH, MD, FAcadMEd, SFHEA
Consultant Paediatrician, Whittington Health, London, UK
and
Course Director UCL iBSc in
Paediatrics and Child Health, London (2010-2016)

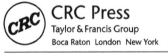

CRC Press
Taylor & Francis Group
Boca Raton London New York

CRC Press is an imprint of the
Taylor & Francis Group, an **informa** business

CRC Press
Taylor & Francis Group
6000 Broken Sound Parkway NW, Suite 300
Boca Raton, FL 33487-2742

International Standard Book Number-13: 978-1-78523-124-7 (Paperback)

Visit the Taylor & Francis Web site at
http://www.taylorandfrancis.com

and the CRC Press Web site at
http://www.crcpress.com

We would like to dedicate this book to all those families who have experienced difficult or painful journeys. We hope that it may go some way to improving journeys for families in the future.

Contents

Foreword

The purpose of a storyteller is not to tell you how to think, but to give you the questions to think upon.

Brandon Sanderson
The Way of Kings

On 12 September 1940, four French teenagers entered a secret passageway which led them to an extraordinary discovery: the first recorded stories. In the Lascaux Caves in the Pyrenees Mountains, they stumbled upon a series of cave paintings dating back to between 15,000 and 13,000 BC. The paintings told their stories through depictions of animals, humans and abstract signs. Storytelling, then, is part of our history and culture, uniquely human and preceding the written word as a way of conveying tradition and belief, happiness and sorrow, victory and defeat, joy and despair. It is a primal part of our being.

This is first and foremost a book of stories; the raw uncut narratives of parents of children with a range of complex conditions. It is a book that provokes, challenges and teaches through this medium. Medical training has long been considered an apprenticeship for one reason alone: doctors, and indeed other healthcare professionals, learn their art not from textbooks, but from people. Knowledge gained from textbooks provides an understanding of the theoretical basis of our clinical world and helps build semantic learning. But it is our episodic memories of individual patient encounters that really embed our knowledge; the way in which a mother touched her husband's hand when we broke some bad news about her child, or the unruly curly hair of the child with severe asthma who was so slow to respond to treatment. I became convinced of the importance of the patient journey as a teaching medium when I was Director of Medical Education at Great Ormond Street Hospital. By replacing the traditional 'Grand Round' with the dramatised story of Daniel – a boy with cystic fibrosis who we 'subjected' to every possible misadventure from drug errors and system failures to ethical issues of consent and personal autonomy – we captured the imagination of the entire hospital. Staff who dealt with the life-and-death rollercoaster of severe illness every day were nonetheless engaged and involved in our fictional dramatisation, discussing how things could have been done differently and better.

This book builds on those same principles, but with the added dimension that these are not fictional stories; they are real accounts, recounted by parents generously prepared to share what in some cases must have been the most harrowing periods of their lives. The stories raise many questions in their own right, but the authors further guide the reader with suggested themes and discussion points.

It is worth mentioning two recurrent themes which illustrate the commonest pitfalls in clinical care: poor communication and poor systems. If only we could get these two aspects of care right, we would be doing the best for our patients, even though we cannot always prolong life or improve clinical outcomes. 'Good communication skills' has become a rather bland descriptor for what our patients need and deserve. It has been said that computers communicate, but humans connect, and I very much hope that readers of this book will learn the importance of 'connection' through a better understanding of what it means to experience both good and bad care from the other side of the fence. However, our frustration when things go wrong despite our best efforts is often down to the complex healthcare environment in which we all work. We are part of a wider system of sometimes quite tortuous processes within our department, hospital or wider clinical network. It often seems like it is impossible to influence these systems when a patient falls through the cracks. I would, however, urge readers of this book to think about how they can improve even a small local system, because by doing so, the next parent travelling the same pathway may have a smoother journey.

Everyone involved in the delivery of healthcare could benefit and gain important insights from reading this book; medical students and doctors, nurses, allied healthcare professionals and service managers. And if as a result there are a few more good stories to tell in the future, then the book will have done its job.

Dr Hilary Cass

*Director of Education and Workforce, Evelina London Children's Hospital
Clinical Advisor, Children's and Young People's Healthcare,
Health Education England*

Acknowledgements

We would like to thank the following individuals for their help and support in the creation of this book: Professor Paul Winyard, Dr Benita Morrisey, Dr Rose Crowley, Caroline Smith and Nike Adigun.

Our contributors are:

Dr Sebastian Kraemer, Former Consultant Psychiatrist, Whittington Health and tutor for UCL iBSc in Paediatrics and Child Health, London, 2010–2016

Dr Hilary Cass, Director of Education and Workforce, Evelina London, and Children's Hospital Clinical Advisor, Children's and Young People's Healthcare, Health Education England

Dr Bryony Alderman (written while a foundation doctor, but previously a student on the iBSc 2010–2011)

Carol Nahra (mother and journalist)

The medical students involved are:

Anna Mullan, Sabie Rainton, Rachel Blackman-Mac, Urvi Patel, Elspeth Bisson, Beth Brockbank, Rebecca Piper, Samuel Gittens, Sara Tho-Calvi, Karishma Desai, Felicity Ockelford, Hansini Sivaguru, Poppy Redman, James Williams, Alex Harper and Shivan Kotecha.

1

How to Use This Book

Chloe Macaulay, Polly Powell and Caroline Fertleman

This book is a collection of stories that represent the journeys of the many families who have children with long-term or complex conditions.

It is not rocket science, and yet it feels as if we are only just beginning to realise that good healthcare is about more than making a diagnosis and giving the correct medical treatment – the *experience* of those going through the system is hugely important. Parents will remember forever how a piece of news was broken, or the nurse who was dismissive when their child said he was hungry, or the one who noticed his team's football shirt that he is so proud of. And communication – communication is absolutely key.

We developed these patient journeys for our undergraduate course in Paediatrics and Child Health as a response to the recognition that not enough emphasis was being placed on the *patient journey* – not only the physical journey through the different professionals, hospitals and organisations that children with severe or complex illnesses have, but also the social and emotional journey. How does it feel to have a 'label' of cerebral palsy? What impact does having a child with a disability have on your ability to work or to get after-school care? How does it affect siblings? We felt that talking to patients and parents about their experiences would not only help our students to develop as reflective, thoughtful clinicians, but would also expose them to the challenges of the system – the obstacle courses that families have to try and navigate themselves.

So we started collecting stories from families, real-life stories of their experiences – some good, some bad. Most are a combination of the two. As we explored these stories with our medical students, we encouraged them to see the experiences from the families' perspective, to put themselves in their shoes – 'How would it feel to be told that your child might die, or to be told you were being irrational?' Several themes emerged time and time again – the importance of communication, the difficult aspects of diagnosis and clinical care, roles and responsibilities, the emotional impact on us of working with children and families, the wider impact of illness and the often confusing organisation of care and services. Our students told us that they found that studying and discussing patient journeys and talking to families gave them a completely different perspective. Because of this, we have tried to make them more widely available in this book.

Although developed for use with medical students (many of these stories have actually been collected by medical students), we feel that these journeys would be useful for anyone working for children with chronic and complex conditions, including nurses and other allied health professionals, as well as psychology students. They are all real – the words of children, parents or family members.

At the end of the book, you will find a short account from one of our students, discussing what exploring these stories has meant to her. We have also included a chapter written by child psychiatrist Dr Sebastian Kraemer, whose insights and experience led to wonderfully rich discussions with the students about the journeys. His chapter helps us to understand the challenges we as individuals face when we step into a patient journey and why it is important to reflect on our experiences. Finally, one of the parents who has kindly allowed us to use her family's story in this book concludes with her thoughts and feelings on why it is important for us all to listen to and reflect on patient journeys.

There is no set way to use this book. We have used the journeys as a focus for discussion in small groups with both a paediatrician and a child psychiatrist, but they can be read alone or used for written assignments. There are lots of different themes or issues that come out of each journey – we have added a suggestion of topics for discussion aligned to the themes that have emerged for our group. This is not by any means an exhaustive list, but is there as a prompt to help get you started. Reading and discussing these stories is only the beginning. We hope that it will encourage you to start having *different* conversations with families and exploring and improving your own patients' journeys.

Thank you to the families who have shared their journeys with us. We hope that many families will have better journeys as a result.

2

Patient Journeys

Chloe Macaulay, Polly Powell and Caroline Fertleman

Most of the names of the children in this book have been changed to protect anonymity. However, David and Dillon's parents wanted their children's real names to be used.

AASIF

When my wife and I first heard she was pregnant, we were so thrilled. For a while, everything was perfect. It was only when Aasif was about 3 years old that we noticed something was wrong. His stomach was very swollen and hard. We were quite concerned – parents' intuition I think – so we took him to the paediatrician at our local hospital. He just brushed aside our concerns and said, 'It's probably gas! Nothing to worry about'.

A week later, we were at an appointment with the physiotherapist about his walking. She noticed his tummy and said, 'This isn't normal, it could be his spleen'. She referred us to another hospital about 40 minutes' drive away. They were great there and everything was dealt with so smoothly. We were happy not to be going back to our first doctor after our past experience. They referred us to the children's hospital within a week. What a difference in service!

At the children's hospital they did every test imaginable. It was a relief to finally be getting somewhere. We went home to wait for the results, but over the next couple of days, Aasif got very ill. He was waking up in the morning, shaking and vomiting. We just wanted to know what was causing it. We were called back to the children's hospital within 3 days for more tests.

Aasif was getting restless by now; it was a lot for a 3 year old to take in. I could tell it was making my wife anxious – she stopped eating or sleeping. I had to keep it together for her and Aasif. The dad is supposed to be the strong one, I guess.

Then the diagnosis was made. It was like a weight had been lifted. The doctor told us Aasif had **glycogen storage disorder type 3**, something very rare. We were told it might have been something to do with the fact that my wife and I are cousins, because of our genes and stuff. We felt very guilty at first, knowing we could have caused this. In our culture, this isn't seen as a problem, and our religion and culture are part of who we are. Given the chance again, I wouldn't do anything differently. We love Aasif so much as he is. It's just the hand you're dealt, God's will. At least that's what I believe.

At 4 years old, Aasif had a **nasogastric tube** fitted to help him with eating. We had an awful time with it. He was so self-conscious going to nursery. He'd get really upset every morning before going and then when he was there he would cry constantly. It was horrible to see him so distressed. We worried about his development too. He'd already been late to start walking, and with all these problems at nursery, we could see him falling even further behind. He's at a mainstream school now and they're doing their best to help us, but we have to accept that it's never going to be enough. We like him being with other kids his age, but we have to be realistic. We're looking into sending him to a special school, but the ones near us are expensive. My wife has had to give up her job and I'm working every hour God sends, so we're struggling as it is.

After a couple of years with the nasogastric tube, we knew something had to be changed. Aasif just wasn't happy. We'd spoken to lots of doctors about a **PEG** before, but I wasn't too sure about it. I did a lot of reading; I had to completely understand what it was and how it worked before he could have it fitted. The doctor arranged for us to talk to a family who had a little boy with a PEG. They told us what a difference it had made for them, and hearing their story reassured me that it was nothing like I had imagined.

Aasif has had the PEG for 4 years now and we've never looked back. What a difference! They taught my wife how to do everything and now she feeds him three times a day. She even goes into his school to give him his 11 o'clock feed. It's a full-time job for her, she's an expert. She can tell when he's going to have low sugar without even testing his bloods.

We used to really worry about his development, but now we're just seeing how it goes. He can't write and his speech and language are quite behind, but we don't like to focus on what he isn't doing yet. Every time he learns a new word or does something new is a little victory. We've learned to adjust our expectations. We try not to compare him to other children his age, what's the point?

We've discussed having more children and we've been offered **genetic counselling**, but at the moment Aasif is our main priority. He needs all our energy and attention right now. We want everything for him; more physiotherapy, more educational help… there's a long list. A sister or brother for him would be wonderful, but if it happens, it happens. We'll just see how it goes…

Journey collected by Anna Mullan, medical student

GLOSSARY

genetic counselling: Families are seen by a Geneticist (a doctor specialising in genes and inherited conditions) and are given advice based on their family history and genetic testing about their risks of passing on conditions to their children. In this case, the parents are cousins and therefore may be at increased risk of passing on conditions that run in the family to their children.

glycogen storage disorder type 3: A rare inherited disorder that can cause build-up of glycogen in the body. This can lead to abnormal functioning of the liver and muscles and to the liver becoming enlarged. There are different types, but children may suffer with low sugar levels and hyperlipidaemia (high fat levels in their blood). They can go on to develop problems with their liver function and liver failure. It is usually managed with a special diet.

nasogastric tube: A plastic tube put through the nostril, down the oesophagus and into the stomach. It can be used to administer nutrition and medicines.

PEG: Percutaneous endoscopic gastrostomy. This is a small tube inserted through the skin of the abdominal wall and into the stomach in order to administer nutrition and medicines directly into the stomach. It is inserted in an operating theatre while the child is asleep.

THEMES FOR DISCUSSION

Information and communication
- Parental intuition

Roles and relationships
- Different family roles
- Family members as carers

Diagnosis and clinical care
- Genetic counselling and testing
- The 'relief' of receiving a definite diagnosis

Wider impact of illness
- How illnesses are perceived in different cultures and religions
- Helping children with medical conditions to integrate

Organisation of care and services
- Financial help available to families
- Special schools

ABBEY

First of all, I should tell you that I'm a **Type 1 diabetic**, but I wasn't diagnosed until after my first pregnancy. Before I became pregnant I experienced some odd changes. I lost about 10 kg and I was really angry and temperamental all the time. We know now that it was the onset of the diabetes, but at the time my partner, and even I, thought I was going crazy.

A few months later I fell pregnant. One day at a routine appointment at 29 weeks, the midwife mentioned to me that I had raised **ketones**. She didn't explain what these were, and sent me home telling me to expect a letter for an appointment. This was in December, so when the letter didn't arrive I thought it was probably due to Christmas delaying everything. I thought that because they hadn't sent me the appointment, it couldn't have been that important.

It wasn't until after the New Year that I realised that something was really wrong. I went into the emergency department at my local hospital and was admitted immediately. I was told that I had developed **gestational diabetes** and that this had caused blot clots to develop in my unborn son's brain and lungs. I lost him later that day.

After that, the doctors told me that I should keep all the appointments that had already been made. I had to go to a gestational diabetes clinic only a few days later. When I came in, they started asking me questions about when the baby was due. No one had thought to let the team know that I had lost the baby; I had to tell them myself. There was a communication problem at that hospital. In fact, there were a lot of communication problems. I was actually even berated by one of the nurses there. She told me that I should have gone straight to hospital when the midwife told me I had raised ketones, and how silly I was to wait for an appointment. I was doing what the midwife had told me to do. I trusted her. How was I supposed to know any different?

There followed a pretty tough few months as I tried to cope with losing my baby and began to lose weight and have mood swings again. Finally, I was diagnosed with Type 1 diabetes and all those days and weeks of feeling unwell began to make sense. A year and a half later I became pregnant again. This time my care was at a different hospital. The doctors decided that with my diabetes, it would be best to induce my pregnancy at 35 weeks, but my waters broke 3 days before the induction date. After I was admitted, a midwife gave me the drugs to induce labour, even though it had already begun. I suppose it was another communication error, but after that everything went crazy. I had what felt like 50 people in the room. They told me I was having an emergency **caesarean section**. The **anaesthetist** couldn't get the **epidural** in. It was just manic, probably the most stressful experience of my entire life. But at the end of it I got a lovely little baby girl, Mia. So I can't really complain, can I?

Compared to that experience, my next baby's birth felt like a breeze. Abbey was delivered by planned caesarean. At 34 weeks into the pregnancy, the doctors felt that they weren't happy with the management of my diabetes, so they decided it was time to get her out. I knew that as she was early at 34 weeks she would be rushed off to check everything was OK, so wasn't surprised when this happened, but it was a bit of a bombshell when they didn't bring her back. Instead, they told us there was something wrong with her bowels. Nothing is ever easy, is it?

We were referred to this specialist hospital and the doctors there were amazing. I remember one doctor in particular was just wonderful. He sat down with us and explained everything. Abbey had a **bowel malrotation**. He drew us diagrams showing us what had happened, and really took his time. His manner was wonderful and he made some light-hearted jokes, which I know really helped to put my partner at ease.

We were given a flat just round the corner so Mia could stay with us while Abbey was in hospital. There are so many people to help you, and everyone is so approachable. I was even given vouchers for food and a private room in which to express milk. We feel we can always bring Mia as well because there are so many play facilities. Mia adores coming here and still talks about the red truck in the **NICU** parents' room.

After Abbey had recovered from the surgery, we were discharged back to the local hospital for 2 weeks. It was very hard going back there; I think I had a bit of a trust issue. Obviously at the specialist hospital you know that the facilities, the doctors, staff and treatments are all the best possible. Also, the atmosphere is so friendly and warm. At the local hospital, everything feels more severe. At the specialist hospital, the baby cots are open top; whereas at the local hospital, the babies are in closed-in incubators. The incubators meant I couldn't easily touch my child, which sounds simple, but is so important to a mother. At the local hospital, they make you leave the room while the staff handover, which makes you feel excluded, whereas at the specialist hospital you are allowed to stay.

On the NICU, you always hear doctors and parents talk about setbacks. Luckily for us, there seemed to be no setbacks. We were able to take Abbey home and it looked like we were in the clear. Unfortunately, last night Abbey experienced a setback. She was vomiting and it was green, just like in her first few days of life. To be honest, I didn't want to do anything about it. Abbey seemed happy, so I thought she was fine. However, my partner didn't agree and I reluctantly let him take her into the local hospital. They called the surgical team here who had performed her operation, and the surgeons wanted her back to check everything was OK. I know my partner made the right decision to bring her in. I think I wasn't quite ready to admit that there might be another problem.

My partner has had a difficult time with all of this. The NICU in some respects is very much a women's domain. At the local hospital especially I don't think he felt welcome. He's Italian, so he's got that whole macho complex going on. I don't blame him, but he's not very open when it comes to discussing our problems. He couldn't even say the name of our son who died out loud until a couple of months ago. My mother is around, but she's very old and doesn't understand what is going on. My partner's mother actually lost two babies herself, so she knows a lot about what I've been through. She's been helpful in explaining what it's like to my partner; he's always a lot more sensitive after he's been on the phone to her. Sadly, she only speaks Italian (which I don't), so it's hard for us to communicate, but I feel there is a bond there despite the lack of words.

Being pregnant with Abbey was very emotionally draining for me. The day the doctors made the decision to deliver her was the anniversary of our son's death. It put me in a very dark place. At points I was utterly convinced I was going to lose her just like I had our son. I must have gone to the local hospital three or four times just because I felt something wasn't right. I turned down counselling previously, but with Abbey's pregnancy, it was time to start. Having someone to talk to was more helpful than I'd imagined. Thanks to the counselling I came through it, and I feel very lucky to have her now.

I think the NHS is a wonderful organisation. The people in it and the job they do are amazing. The specialist centre is outstanding, but it has a great deal of funding behind it to ensure it is that way. The first hospital we went to, on the other hand, was understaffed and very stretched. Looking back over my experience, I know that mistakes have been made. I realise now that that midwife should have sent me straight to hospital. Sometimes I wonder whether if I had pushed the doctors to let me keep Abbey cooking in me a little longer, then maybe she wouldn't have had a bowel malrotation. But there's no point in wallowing. The way I look at it, maybe losing my son was supposed to happen… I don't blame anyone. After all, you can't blame a human for only being human.

Journey collected by Rachel Blackman-Mac, medical student

GLOSSARY

anaesthetist: A doctor who specialises in providing anaesthetics for patients (putting them to sleep with a general anaesthetic for major procedures or providing pain relief such as epidurals when appropriate). They may also have expertise in pain control and intensive care.

bowel malrotation: When a baby is born with an abnormally rotated gut. The intestine starts off as a long, straight tube and, as it grows and develops, it has to curl up in the correct way to fit inside the baby's abdomen. If it does not curl up correctly, this is called a malrotation. Malrotation can lead to the bowel twisting on itself, cutting off its own blood supply and causing obstruction of the bowel. A baby with malrotation may present with abdominal distention and bilious vomiting (bringing up green bile) and requires an urgent surgical assessment and possible operation.

caesarean section: An operation by which a baby is delivered surgically via an incision to the mother's abdomen. It may be done as a planned procedure or as an emergency for a number of reasons relating to both mother and baby.

epidural: A procedure in which an anaesthetic is administered through a needle into an area of the spine known as the epidural space and numbs the spinal nerves, causing numbness of the body below the level of injection. This may be used to provide pain relief for a procedure such as caesarean section, without the need to put the woman to sleep.

gestational diabetes: A form of diabetes that comes on during pregnancy. In many cases, the woman will need treatment during pregnancy, but her blood sugar levels usually improve once she has given birth and may just require monitoring.

ketones: A source of energy produced by the breakdown of fat in the body. Normally, our body uses sugar as a source of energy to allow us to function day to day. However, in diabetes, the body cannot utilise the sugar properly and therefore has to break down fat into ketones as an alternative source of energy. A high level of ketones in the body (detected in urine or blood) is an indicator that the diabetes is not being well controlled (often seen in newly diagnosed diabetics) and can cause diabetic ketoacidosis.

NICU: Neonatal intensive care unit, where specialist care is provided for newborn babies who are unwell or premature and in need of support.

Type 1 diabetic: Diabetes is a condition in which there is abnormal sugar control in the body, leading to abnormally high sugar levels in the blood. This can cause weight loss, thirst, increase in passing urine and, when uncontrolled, can lead to a dangerous situation called diabetic ketoacidosis. There are different types of diabetes. Broadly, Type 1 diabetes is due to inadequate production of insulin by the pancreas in the body, Type 2 diabetes is associated with lifestyle and weight and gestational diabetes is brought on in pregnancy. Insulin is a hormone in the body that controls sugar levels in order to maintain a healthy balance. The treatment of Type 1 diabetes is insulin in the form of daily injections, which are needed for life. Diet must also be controlled.

THEMES FOR DISCUSSION

Information and communication
- Advantages and disadvantages of different types of communication (e.g. lost letters, telephone calls etc.)
- Failure to communicate important information – why this might happen

Roles and relationships
- Trust
- Being a father vs. being a mother (e.g. in the NICU)

Diagnosis and clinical care
- Missing a diagnosis – why this might happen and how it could be dealt with

Wider impact of illness
- Effect of stillbirth/miscarriage
- How different people deal with loss

Organisation of care and services
- How different hospitals work (e.g. allowing parents to be present while staff handover the patients vs. asking them to leave)

ASHOKA

It wasn't her fault. My mum had a normal pregnancy and I was born healthy. There was no reason to think that I was suffering from something serious. It all began in Sri Lanka when I was 3 years old. I kept complaining of tummy aches and it hurt every time I went to wee. We lived in a small village, so if we needed to see a doctor, we had to make a carefully planned trip to the capital. We only visited a doctor when we knew that we had no other choice. I was too young to realise that I needed medical attention sooner. I suffered for a year before we sought help.

The doctor told my mum that I had something called a **hernia**, which was causing the pain. She sent us home within minutes. I don't think my mum even understood the doctor's explanation. Despite this, she accepted what she was told. The pain worsened and my mum continued to ignore my complaints. In her eyes, we had an answer and that was that. Eventually I had to go back to hospital, when I started screaming from the pain.

At the second visit, another doctor told us that we would be better off seeing doctors in a developed country, where they could perform more specialised tests. Although Sri Lanka provides free healthcare, the hospital didn't have the resources I needed. This doctor left my mother with a life-changing choice to make. We already knew other families who had moved abroad successfully. It took 5 years for my parents to make a decision. We finally packed our bags and moved to the UK in search of medical help.

Our whole family moved. My siblings and I had to leave our school and our friends behind and my dad had to find a new job. After I arrived in the UK, I was referred by the GP to my local hospital. They explained that they couldn't help me either, so they sent me to the children's hospital. There, the doctors and nurses did lots of scans and tests to find the cause of my problem.

Eventually, a urodynamic test showed that the flow of urine from my kidneys was blocked. At the age of 9, I was told that my symptoms were caused by a problem called **hydronephrosis**. Hearing the doctor explain this meant that I could finally blame my symptoms on something real; however, at the same time I felt frustrated. I wished that I had been able to come to the children's hospital straightaway. No one was able to give us a definite answer until then.

The **nephrologist** told me I would have to learn how to **self-catheterise** in order to help the urine flow out of my body. It was tough for me as I was young, and being in hospital in a new country was a big shock. The nurses taught me how to self-catheterise when I was 9 because I couldn't come into hospital every time I needed to wee. At school, it was hard when my friends asked me why I was in the boys' toilets for so long. Looking back, having to learn how to care for myself at that age meant that I had to grow up quickly and become independent.

By the time I turned 12, the nephrologist explained that I would need a kidney transplant before my 18th birthday. A million questions went through my head – questions I still don't know the answer to. All I knew was that my future had been set. I needed to look after my kidneys as best as I could until the chance for a transplant came up.

The constant check-ups and appointments became the normality in my life. I stopped worrying, as I had been managing my catheterisation well and wasn't experiencing any of the previous pain. One afternoon at an appointment, my doctor looked at me. I can still remember the worry in his eyes. He explained that both my kidneys were so badly damaged that I would need a transplant as soon as possible, even though I was 15. Everything came 3 years earlier than I was expecting. It all happened so quickly. I was immediately put on the waiting list for a kidney and so the waiting game began.

The Waiting Game

I don't know why my mum didn't want to donate her kidney to me. So whilst I waited for a kidney donor, I was put on **peritoneal dialysis**. I had to be trained for this again. I learnt medical skills that helped to keep me healthy. In a way, it was just like learning how to tie my shoelaces. But with shoelaces, if you don't do them up properly, the worst outcome is that you may trip and graze yourself. With dialysis, I had to be careful I didn't get an infection that could make me very ill. Following months of continuous infections, I was transferred to **haemodialysis**. Both were just as bad as each other. I had to sleep with peritoneal dialysis every night for 9 hours, but I could stay at home. On the other hand, with haemodialysis, I had to come into hospital four times a week. It was easier to manage as the nurses did everything for me and my mum didn't have to come with me, but I still missed lots of school.

A year passed as I continued to wait. In that time, the longest period of school I was able to attend consecutively was for 6 weeks. My grades were affected and the doctors had to tell my school because of my frequent absences. They were very understanding, but my friends weren't. They couldn't understand how ill I was. I didn't want to tell them that I needed a kidney transplant because I didn't want them to feel sorry for me.

Eventually, my mum agreed to donate a kidney to me. I think she changed her mind when I fainted during an afternoon of dialysis. We had to go through many rigorous tests to make sure that my mum was a match. This was an extremely difficult time for my family. My dad had to take a lot of time off work to take my mum to the hospital for testing. This meant that my three siblings missed school because no one was there to pick them up and drop them off. It was also a time of financial hardship, as my parents were unable to work.

When they phoned to tell us that my mum was a match, I didn't know what to say. At first, I didn't want to take her kidney. This was my problem and so I felt that I needed to face it alone. I felt guilty for what she had to do for me. Both our lives were going to change. Later on, after I accepted the reality of the situation, I had to be taken off the waiting list for a kidney. It was only then that I found out that I had never been put on the waiting list due to a system error.

The children's hospital doesn't treat adults, so my mum had to have her kidney removed at a different hospital. On the day of the operation, she wasn't there with me. My uncle kept me company because my dad stayed with my mum. I was more worried about my mum than myself. She was so far away and I couldn't find out how she was doing.

Life Post-Transplant

I felt immediately better after receiving the transplant. I was a lot less tired. My mum and dad couldn't spend a lot of time with me while I was recovering because they had to look after my younger siblings. I always slept in the hospital alone. Soon, I was allowed to go home and return to school. I had missed so much that I had to redo Year 12 at a different school. All the students in my year thought I was a retake and looked down on me. When I told them I had had a kidney transplant, they thought I was lying. You couldn't tell just by looking at me.

It's a year on, now, and I've never felt better. I'm more active and the doctors have told me that my new kidney will last a lifetime as long as I look after it. The transplant has made such a difference. When I was 15, I used to have to take over 21 tablets throughout the day. Now I have to take ten. I just have to remember to take them at the right times.

What Lies Ahead?

I will soon be moving to the adult kidney services at a different hospital. It will be hard. Everyone here knows my story. I don't know anyone there and I will miss all of the kind nurses who I have gotten to know.

This experience has inspired me to become a doctor, perhaps even a nephrologist. People always ask me if I am angry that the doctors in Sri Lanka couldn't help. I'm not upset about it. My parents are angry, but now I'm better and that's what matters. My condition is my problem to deal with and I don't want other people to treat me differently. In a way, I've learnt so much because of it. I never feel like it shouldn't have happened.

Journey collected by Urvi Patel, medical student

GLOSSARY

haemodialysis: Dialysis is the filtering of waste products and excess water from the blood. This is a job that is done by the kidneys, so dialysis is required when the kidneys are not functioning adequately. In haemodialysis, blood is removed from the body and filtered in a special haemodialysis machine to remove the unwanted products, before being returned to the body. This needs to be done in a specialist unit and will typically happen three or four times a week and takes around 4 hours each time.

hernia: This occurs when an internal part of the body pushes through a weakness in the muscle wall of the body. For example, an umbilical hernia occurs when underlying bowel or fatty tissue pushes through a weakness in the abdominal wall.

hydronephrosis: Meaning 'water in the kidney'; this refers to swelling and dilatation of the inside of the kidney due to build-up of urine. This can occur when there is a blockage to the flow of urine out of the kidneys.

nephrologist: A doctor who specialises in diseases of the kidney.

peritoneal dialysis: This is another type of dialysis which involves the use of the peritoneum, a membrane that lines the abdominal cavity, as a kind of filter through which the waste products can be removed. A special fluid is put into the peritoneal cavity and the body absorbs the things it needs from the fluid and excretes the things it does not need into the fluid through the membrane using a peritoneal dialysis machine. This can be done at home overnight while the patient is sleeping.

self-catheterisation: Urethral catheterisation is where a tube is inserted through the urethra up into the bladder to allow the drainage of urine. Most commonly this is performed by a doctor or nurse, but it can also be performed by the patient at home ('self-catheterisation'). This may be necessary when the patient is unable to pass urine, most commonly due to a blockage, but it is undesirable to have a permanent catheter in place. Therefore, when the patient needs to pass urine, they can pass a catheter to allow the bladder to drain. This needs to be done aseptically to prevent infection.

THEMES FOR DISCUSSION

Information and communication
- Checking understanding

Roles and relationships
- Accepting doctors' reassurances
- Taking responsibility for yourself
- Parents as organ donors for their children

Diagnosis and clinical care
- Diagnostic tests available in different places

Wider impact of illness
- Migration for health reasons
- Accepting a new normality
- Effect on friendships

Organisation of care and services
- Healthcare in developing countries
- Transition to adult services

AVA

Oh no, we're not Mum and Dad. I'm Nan, and this is my friend Steve.

Ava has **septo-optic dysplasia**. My three children, including Ava's dad, never had any health problems. I'd never even heard of her condition until she was diagnosed. It doesn't come from anyone – 18 months of genetic testing and nothing came back. It's just God's way that Ava is how she is.

When Ava was 6 weeks old, I noticed her eyes didn't follow movements. It took some persuading before her mum finally took her to the doctors. They said it was just a squint and told us not to worry. I knew this wasn't right and, as I began to spend more time with Ava, I realised other things weren't right either.

Ava's always had problems with food. She is three and a half and still only takes baby formula milk. We can get her to eat some baby food from jars, but only if it is completely pureed. We've tried really hard to introduce even tiny lumps, but our Ava refuses – she just won't eat it. Therapists at school are trying too, but it's a struggle.

When I was looking after Ava, I realised she wasn't digesting things properly. After taking her to hospital four or five times, somebody finally listened to me. Ava was whisked from her local hospital to the specialist children's hospital for more tests. This is when we got her diagnosis. Around this time, Ava was put into foster care.

Ava had two lovely sets of foster parents, but it was the second family that properly encouraged her. That's when she really started to develop. I was allowed to keep in touch. At first I saw her every Tuesday evening, then every weekend. She's lived with me permanently for just over a year, and 2 weeks ago I finally got official **guardianship**. It was a long struggle and lots of paperwork, but she's worth the effort. Her foster carers are in touch over the phone and I take her to see her dad and sometimes her mum – I want her to know her whole family.

It's tiring looking after Ava. I'm lucky though. She's only nursery age and she's already at school 4 days a week. She loves school. They pick her up in the bus at 8 a.m. and drop her back to my house by 4 p.m. It's amazing. I have never missed an appointment for Ava's health, but I feel really bad that I couldn't go to her parents' evening. I don't drive and I can't take Ava on the Tube, we'd both get scared. I hate heights and the escalators are fundamentally dangerous. Every day her school and I fill in report cards. These describe what Ava's been enjoying, doing well at or struggling with. Ava hates change. If everybody knows what's happening, then we can make sure she gets as little disruption as possible. School has helped her so much. They have a whole **multidisciplinary team** to support her when she's there. It's so much easier now it's all in one place.

Blindness is common with septo-optic dysplasia. It's not Ava's eyes that are damaged – they're bright and blue and beautiful. But she can't see. She will never see. I was told that there is a problem with her nerve endings for sight and her brain can't process the information. Ava's registered with a specialist eye hospital in London. We don't really see much of them because they can't do anything. It's best if someone who can be helped gets her appointment.

Ava's an incredibly resourceful child. She has only been to Steve's house three times and already pretty much knows her way around. She uses her feet to reach and feel in front of her then shuffles with her bum and hands. She uses touch to familiarise herself and remember the furniture. I tried blindfolding myself to see how Ava feels – it was scary and impossible to move around and, unlike Ava, I'd already seen the room before I was blindfolded.

Ava can sing you the whole Top 40. Her hearing is great and she's good at recognising rhythm and tunes. She loves music as it comforts her and keeps her calm and happy. Ava recognises people by their voices – her head always turns when I speak to her. I'm worried that she isn't talking yet. She started seeing a **speech and language therapist** a few months ago; they said she is like a 9 month old, making noises but no words. Somebody told me that it's probably **autism** because lots of children with septo-optic dysplasia have this. Her school disagrees. I haven't had a chance to research autism yet.

Ava's doing well. I can tell that she is constantly learning and developing. Her growth hormone injections mean that she's catching up in size too. She's actually getting so big she's a handful and I'm constantly buying new clothes! I think Ava may need treatment for the rest of her life. But we're here, we're managing, and that's much better than not having realised anything was wrong.

Journey collected by Elspbeth Bisson, medical student

GLOSSARY

autism: A complex disorder of brain development which affects communication, social interaction and behaviour to varying degrees.

guardianship: The legal guardian of a child is responsible for the child's safety and wellbeing. The decision to make someone a legal guardian is made by the court following an assessment by social services.

multidisciplinary team: A team made up of people from various professional backgrounds with different expertise within healthcare. For example, a paediatrician, ward sister, occupational therapist, physiotherapist, dietician and psychologist might meet to discuss a patient.

septo-optic dysplasia: A rare condition in which a child is born with two or more of the following: abnormal development of the optic nerve; abnormal development of the midline structures of the brain; and/or abnormalities of the pituitary gland.

speech and language therapist: A professional who specialises in assessing speech, language, communication and swallowing.

THEMES FOR DISCUSSION

Information and communication
- Sources of information

Roles and relationships
- Importance of establishing who the carer is

Diagnosis and clinical care
- Sensory impairment

Organisation of care and services
- Multidisciplinary team
- Looked-after children
- Special schools

DAVID

When we received the devastating news that my only son, David Anderson Davis, had cancer on 4th July 2013, the diagnosis was impossible to comprehend.

This shock diagnosis followed months of visits to the A&E department of our local hospital as David had persistently suffered with fairly mild, but nevertheless unexplainable nosebleeds. As David was clinically a very 'well' and energetic child with a healthy appetite, it was at this time almost impossible not to believe that an incorrect diagnosis had been made.

Following a quick referral to our local cancer centre, David's consultant contacted me saying he didn't believe the diagnosis of **nasopharyngeal carcinoma** was correct, mentioning a possibility of his tumour being **benign**, and David's scheduled treatment was postponed pending further investigation: a **PET scan** and surgery. Whilst awaiting the promised call for surgery, the extremely aggressive nature of David's illness became horrifically apparent.

The tumour visibly grew at an alarming rate, obstructing David's breathing. When the telephone call failed to materialise, I rushed him to the A&E department of a hospital where I knew the correct surgeons to perform the operation David desperately needed were based. By this point, David's blood pressure had also become alarmingly high. We anxiously waited for his notes to be transferred to the hospital and a slot for surgery was eventually booked for Tuesday 6th August.

During the afternoon of Friday 2nd August, David began haemorrhaging uncontrollably, and the tumour by this time had grown outside of his nose to the size of a huge plum. Emergency life-saving surgery was performed around midnight, along with a blood transfusion, and David was kept in the **PICU** over the weekend.

The following Thursday, we were told that David's condition was terminal, that the tumour was now sitting directly under the membrane of his brain and that it would never respond to treatment.

The following afternoon, David had an operation for the insertion of a **Hickman line** and **nasogastric tube** and we were transferred to the cancer centre for treatment to commence. Following these events, I didn't hesitate to sign the consent forms for **chemotherapy**, but was baffled at the fact that this was the very same treatment plan that had been postponed 3 weeks previously.

During a visit from the consultant days later, we were told that David's condition was one of 40 cases worldwide; however, he urged us to forget the horrific events of the last 2 weeks, to maintain a positive attitude and told me that my actions had saved David's life.

David had three cycles of chemotherapy followed by 6 weeks of combined chemotherapy and **radiotherapy**. Although he suffered from traumatic side effects, including **mucositis** and a blood clot, each and every scan revealed a significant response to treatment.

Following completion of his treatment, David made a remarkably quick recovery and a biopsy taken on 1st April revealed that my son had achieved the impossible and was in **remission**.

Heartbreakingly, however, from May, David began to experience new and worrying symptoms, including aching legs, fevers, back pain and a dry cough, which persisted on and off with vomiting episodes. Each time I reported these I was given various explanations including a possible vitamin D deficiency, a virus and that these were delayed side effects of his radiotherapy treatment and of the blood clot detected the previous November. Having been blocked from getting David examined via the **oncology ward** due to him being 6 months clear of treatment in June of 2014, the paediatric doctor of our local A&E department told me David had a virus and, witnessing my anxiety, told me I needed to accept that he was in remission. His up-to-date head and neck scans had also confirmed this.

A month after this, David developed **tinnitus** and, alarm bells ringing, I took him back to see the paediatrician. She examined David and sent him for a chest X-ray. The X-ray showed what appeared to be disease in his lungs. On 4th July 2014, it was confirmed that the disease had spread to David's lungs, the cavity between his right lung and heart and to his liver. The tumours were now affecting the function of his heart and David was transferred to the PICU. When presented with David's awful prognosis, the consultant asked what was going through my mind. My only response was 'getting the fight back'. I could not entertain the thought of losing my precious son for a single moment.

David's new treatment began that evening, and once again the positive effects of this were immediate. Within a couple of days, David's breathing improved, he was transferred to the oncology ward of the hospital and we were able to return home towards the end of July. The following month, David began to suffer chest symptoms and it was confirmed at the beginning of September that the disease had built up immunity to the treatment.

Long periods of hospital admissions were clearly contributing to David's deterioration and he was no longer eating. When urged to take him home with a prescription for oral chemotherapy, I was too exhausted and distressed to challenge this advice.

Once we returned home, I instantly began to research alternative treatments. I read that traditional Chinese medicine had been found to be beneficial alongside chemotherapy. My plan was to build David up with a combination of my chosen supplements and nutritious food so that by his next scheduled appointment he would be strong enough for me to request the aggressive treatment I knew was needed to tackle this aggressive disease. Initially, David thrived and even gained enough strength to ride his bike again.

Within weeks, however, the horrific impact that this untreated disease was having on David's health became increasingly apparent and I cannot articulate how distressing this was. Witnessing my son's pain, breathless episodes and dependency on oxygen, I instantly regretted not questioning what I had been advised was the best option.

During my frantic calls to the community support team, I was told that nothing could be done until the next appointment at the hospital. David's deterioration was visibly distressing to the consultant by the time the appointment arrived, and a combination of oral/intravenous chemotherapy was scheduled to commence the following Monday.

As this treatment had been mentioned alongside the strongly advised oral chemotherapy the previous month, I expressed my lack of faith in this medicine and questioned its effectiveness. The response I received was shocking. I was basically told to get real and that I was pushing things too far. The consultant then spun his computer screen containing David's chest X-ray towards me. This is the consultant who had always urged me to remain positive and had reassured me of David's remission when I had reported various symptoms in June.

Upon my request, David was admitted onto the ward for the 5-day treatment as he was too weak to make the daily commute. The following day, we were taken to a room by the team to be told that, should David stop breathing, 'we would not trip over ourselves to resuscitate him'.

That Friday, when an ambulance collected David and I for the journey home, I was told in a cryptic way that if David was still alive the following Monday, we should return to the ward for further treatment.

David's health improved so much over the following month that his oxygen requirement decreased from a flow of 10 litres per minute down to 2 litres, and eventually he only depended on this during the night. Having always had a passion for trains, David became well enough to live his dream on 21st November, when he rode on the London Underground system.

Towards the end of November, I was given the shocking news that the disease had continued to progress. This time when I begged his consultant to find another treatment he did not hesitate, and after consulting a hospital in Boston, the new treatment plan meant we were able to enjoy our last precious Christmas with David.

At the beginning of January, David's **central line** became obstructed, and any decisions for further treatment were taken away.

David passed away in my arms at home on 25th January 2015.

Whilst living through the relentless heartbreak of losing my beautiful son, who was also my best friend, I am constantly haunted by the lack of support in the periods outside of David's treatment. On reflection, I faced a constant battle to be listened to from the beginning. I was commended at the beginning for having his diagnosis established at such an early stage, then for not listening to the advice to await a telephone call for surgery, then for pushing to have his relapse diagnosed. I have also recently openly been told by David's consultant that each decision I made regarding treatment was the correct one and that the reason he didn't hesitate to agree to my request for finding his last treatment plan was because he could see that both David and I were not giving up without a fight. He now agrees that the benefits of active treatment by far outweighed the horrific effects of the disease.

Journey written by David's mother

GLOSSARY

benign: Not cancerous.

central line: A form of long-term intravenous access which allows the patient to be given medication through the veins without the repeated need for cannulas. There are different types, including a Hickman line (see below) or portocath.

chemotherapy: A combination of drugs that are used for the treatment of cancer. There are a wide variety of types of chemotherapy, which target cancerous cells in different ways. All have side effects which vary dependent on the type of drug, but may include hair loss, nausea and vomiting.

Hickman line: This central line is a long, thin tube made of silicone rubber that is inserted through one of the veins, usually in the neck, and ends in a large blood vessel near the heart. A small part of the tube will be visible at the neck, through which bloods can be taken or medication administered. In children, this will be put in while they are asleep under anaesthetic.

mucositis: Inflammation of the lining of the mouth and gut. This is a common side effect of some types of chemotherapy and can be very painful, making it difficult to eat and drink.

nasogastric tube: A plastic tube put through the nostril, down the oesophagus and into the stomach. It can be used to administer nutrition and medicines.

nasopharyngeal carcinoma: A type of cancer involving the nose and pharynx (part of the throat just below the nasal cavity). It causes a tumour (growth) within the nasopharynx and may be treated with surgery, chemotherapy and radiotherapy.

oncology ward: A ward for patients with cancer.

PET scan: A type of imaging test in which a special substance is injected into the patient, which is taken up by the tissues of the body in different amounts depending on how much sugar they use. Areas of the body using up large amounts of energy will glow brightly on the scan, and this can be useful to identify certain types of cancer in the body, as cancerous cells are very active. The image will be interpreted by an expert.

PICU: Paediatric intensive care unit.

radiotherapy: A form of treatment used for certain types of cancer which involves firing beams of high-energy radiation ('irradiation') at the tumour. Side effects are common and include soreness of the skin and damage to the areas adjacent to the tumour.

remission: Can be complete or partial. Complete remission refers to the state in which there is no identifiable cancer in the body following treatment, whereas partial indicates the cancer has reduced or has stopped growing.

tinnitus: A persistent ringing in the ears.

THEMES FOR DISCUSSION

Information and communication
- Breaking bad news

Roles and relationships
- Support for cancer patients
- The parent's role as advocate for the child

Diagnosis and clinical care
- Cancer treatment
- Aggressive versus palliative treatment – when to stop
- Do Not Resuscitate orders

Wider impact of illness
- 'Not giving up'

Organisation of care and services
- Palliative care services

DILLON

Dillon was born after a short labour. He was scrawny looking with a big head. A few hours later, his breathing grew erratic, seemingly because he had inhaled **meconium** during the birth. We were transferred to a neonatal ward, where a doctor noticed that Dillon's head looked too large and requested an ultrasound. This showed that his **ventricles** were enlarged. The next day, at less than 48 hours old, Dillon underwent an **EEG** and an **MRI**. The diagnosis was devastating: **polymicrogyria**, meaning 'too many folds'. The condition meant that Dillon's brain had not developed correctly in the womb – completely incorrectly. Cases of polymicrogyria lie on a huge spectrum of seriousness and it seemed Dillon was at the tragic end.

Thus began our intense immersion into hospital life. Our 2 weeks in neonatal were the first in my life I'd spent with nurses. How well I managed to get through each day depended largely on who Dillon's nurse was during any given shift. While Dillon was still at our local hospital, we made the first of many visits to the specialist children's hospital. After looking at Dillon's MRI scans, the consultants shook their heads solemnly and said we should take him home and stimulate him as much as possible.

What we didn't realise during those early weeks was the extent to which Dillon would suffer from **epilepsy**. His first observed **seizure** was when he was a day old in the neonatal ward. Because doctors quickly put him on **phenobarbital**, we did not see him have a seizure until he was living at home with us, and I gradually began to realise that the funny sounds and eye movements that he made were probably fits.

At 2 months, he was readmitted to the children's ward to attempt to get more control over his seizures. He was there for months. With Dillon now on the ward, we slowly became part of an entirely new community, which was to become invaluable to us. Initially, it took a while for us to get to know the different nurses and play specialists, and for them to get to know us. Then my partner came home one day and reported that one of the nurses had confided to him that she loved looking after Dillon, and always asked to do so. We were amazed; someone liked our Dillon. He was not like any other baby on the ward, but he was liked. It was a real boost.

In July, we took Dillon for a day visit to our specialist hospital. Alarmed by his condition, the hospital staff decided to admit him for an extended period. This was a big relief to us because it addressed another of our frustrations: the hospital that controlled Dillon's medication did not really know him. After Dillon had been at the specialist hospital for 2 weeks, a consultant sat us down and told us that they now had a good sense of his condition: Dillon's seizures were intractable, he said, and in his experience, children like Dillon often didn't see their first birthday. The consultant said we could take him to a nearby hospice, essentially to wait for him to die.

However, no such nearby hospice existed. We were distraught. While one part of me wanted him home, another part didn't. So we returned to our local hospital. The ward welcomed us back with open arms; word had been spread that, this time, we would be staying indefinitely. It was an enormous relief to be greeted so warmly. I was so grateful to our local hospital for the wonderful home they provided for Dillon that I became determined to be a model patient's mum: to get on with everyone and never to be a pain.

He didn't pass any major milestones, but he did respond to voices, often by licking his lips. On good days, he could lick and suck, and once we realised this, I encouraged his nursing team to feed him as many lollipops as he liked and made another 'Things that Dillon likes' sign for the wall. After an autumn of relative calm, the winter was long and difficult. Dillon suffered recurring chest infections and, in January, his seizures worsened. He began to have full-blown, **tonic–clonic fits**, which depleted his oxygen levels and made his heart race. He became clearly distressed. With the help of the community **palliative care team**, who were now responsible for guiding Dillon's care, we took the decision to throw out protocols and simply increase his dosage of phenobarbital – the only medicine to which he had ever responded – until his fits stopped. He soon was on four times the normal dose for his weight, and although the visible fits stopped, he was asleep almost all of the time.

In the middle of the night, Dillon died in my arms. He went very peacefully; a quiet end to a turbulent life. As the shifts changed, and we stayed with his body, the nurses going off shift came in to say goodbye. We all cried together. Finally, we walked down to the morgue with two nurses, all four of us crying.

Post Script

Looking back, the single thing which would have improved our lives during our time with Dillon would have been to have had some kind of family key worker. Had someone been assigned to our family who would have helped us negotiate the many different consultations we had every week, both in and outside of hospital, and helped us figure out the best way to proceed on a daily basis, it would have been a godsend. We had a wonderful local hospital, but nonetheless navigating the complex medical and social services terrain we abruptly found ourselves in was difficult and exhausting. We had scores of medical staff looking after us, yet often felt alone. When we found ourselves in hospital for an appointment which turned into hours, then days, then weeks and months, it would have been invaluable if we'd been assigned someone to help us navigate our new world – to be a buffer, a guide, a friend, and to help us see the forest through the trees.

Journey based on writings by Carol Nahra, Dillon's mother

GLOSSARY

EEG: Electroencephalogram; a test used to investigate seizures. Small probes are placed over the head and an electrical tracing of brain activity is taken.

epilepsy: A disorder of the nervous system associated with seizures.

meconium: Sticky black baby stool that looks like tar. Babies normally pass it in the first few days of life, but can sometimes pass it inside the womb before they are born, particularly if they are in distress. Occasionally, they can inhale some into their lungs and this can cause them to have breathing difficulty after birth.

mRI: Magnetic resonance imaging; a type of scan that uses a large magnet to create detailed images of the subject (in this case, the brain).

palliative care team: A team of professionals who specialise in supporting end-of-life care. They can help to control symptoms that may be distressing to the patient, such as pain or seizures.

phenobarbital: A type of barbiturate, which is a medicine used for seizure control.

polymicrogyria: A severe neurological disorder of brain development in which the brain has an excessive number of folds (or 'gyri') on its surface. Children born with this condition can suffer from a variety of different problems, including severe developmental delay and intractable seizures.

seizure: Also known as a *fit*; a seizure is caused by abnormal electrical activity in the brain and can manifest in a number of different ways, including abnormal movements, usually jerking (tonic–clonic seizure), or sometimes stiffness or stillness.

tonic–clonic fit: A type of seizure in which the person is unconscious and the body repeatedly tenses and relaxes, making the person appear to jerk or shake.

ventricles: Fluid-filled spaces in the brain.

THEMES FOR DISCUSSION

Information and communication
- Breaking bad news
- Communication between teams

Roles and relationships
- Dealing with different teams
- The parent as advocate
- Emotional attachment of staff

Diagnosis and clinical care
- The journey to a diagnosis

Wider impact of illness
- Impact on families

Organisation of care and services
- End-of-life care

ELLA

The journey begins. We were in our local hospital for a week before coming here to the children's hospital. During the last week of term before Christmas, Ella started experiencing pain in her legs, which got progressively worse. Then her arms began to ache. Essentially, she could barely move from the waist down. That's how it was.

We went to the local GP who said it was growing pains. Everyone said it was growing pains. We persevered a little and got an appointment to take bloods just after the New Year. I just thought, no, something's not right; we need to get this sorted out.

We managed to get an appointment at the hospital walk-in clinic at silly o'clock on a Saturday night. I don't think the doctor knew what Ella had, but we were brought straight to the paediatric ward. The local hospital didn't do many tests. They performed an **MRI** and took bloods, but that's it.

At day two or three, we saw a consultant with an interest in **rheumatology**. He suggested it could be this 'JDM, blah blah blah… you might have to go to the children's hospital… blah blah blah'. I didn't really think anything more of it. The next day we were told we were waiting for a bed to send Ella to the children's hospital.

We were transferred to the rheumatology ward in the first week of January. There were lots of tests, lots of people prodding and poking. A biopsy was taken, lots of bloods, lots of needles were stuck in her. It was confirmed she had JDM. That meant three lots of medications plus weekly **steroid** injections. She's alright, but she doesn't like needles. I suppose you're in the lap of the gods anyway, aren't you?

You can walk for miles in our favourite park, and in the first week of December we did just that. We walked for 3 hours together; a week later, she's like this. It happened so quickly. Perhaps it had been brewing for a while, and we just didn't know.

Some other children here also have JDM. You see other parents around, but they don't seem to want to talk about it. I'm very open, and I think it would be good to talk. I try not to too much, but it's very easy to Google things too.

We were told in quite a blasé way that she has an enlarged liver – as if saying it would rain tomorrow. They brushed it off as if it's nothing to worry about. But it is; she's my child and I don't want her to have anything wrong. The doctors have a different idea of what is serious and what is not.

During the first week, I'd often ask questions about things. We weren't rudely shut down, but I did soon learn that there was no point in asking. They'd just say we need to do this first or they didn't know.

We very rarely see the doctor. He was around one Saturday morning. There can't be many patients on this ward, but it wasn't until 7 o'clock that evening that we saw him. Maybe he was busy with other things, you don't know, but the nurses are good. The **physio** has more or less told me what the doctors will be telling me today. Should that have come from the physio?

Things also take forever. They'll come in and say we need to do a blood test, but it only happens 3 hours later. By then she's up the wall because she knows she'll be having bloods taken. I think the doctors and nurses should come in when they've got the time, and do whatever they have to there and then. That's my only bugbear at the moment.

The local hospital told us that we'd only be here for a week. Three weeks later, we're still on the ward and they're saying it'll be a minimum of 8 weeks. She is the main priority. However, I do think it's quite nice that some people ask me how I am and if I've eaten; they don't have to.

I'm now signed off work for stress; it's the only way I can get the time off I need. My partner Mike can't take the time off, and I don't want him to, although I haven't seen him in 2 weeks. We don't like to look too far into the future, but he'll need the days off for when Ella eventually comes home.

I give Ella some of her medication now. I don't know how I would cope if I had to give her weekly injections though. From a selfish point of view, I wouldn't want her to associate that pain with me. Bless her, though, I've had to hold her down so many times now in the past 4 weeks, but she always forgives me.

Sadly, things take time. There isn't any magic wand that's going to make Ella better. So yeah.

Journey collected by Beth Brockbank, medical student

GLOSSARY

JDM: Juvenile dermatomyositis; an autoimmune condition (in which the body's immune system attacks healthy tissue) causing inflammation of the muscles, skin and blood vessels. Children often present with a facial rash and muscle weakness. It requires a multidisciplinary team approach and the main treatment is with steroids. The condition can be chronic and very variable in its severity.

MRI: Magnetic resonance imaging; a type of scan that uses a large magnet to create detailed images of the subject (in this case, Ella's joints).

physio: Physiotherapist; a professional who specialises in supporting patients with their physical needs; for example, building up strength and improving mobility.

rheumatology: Specialising in joints, muscles, bones and the immune system.

steroids: Medication used to decrease inflammation. It can be given in a number of different ways; for example, orally, topically (as a cream or ointment) or as an injection.

THEMES FOR DISCUSSION

Information and communication
- Use of jargon/acronyms (e.g. JDM)
- The internet as a source of information

Roles and relationships
- Listening to parents

Diagnosis and clinical care
- The hospital experience

Wider impact of illness
- Losing your identity as a person
- Impact on parents (e.g. stress and prolonged separation)

Organisation of care and services
- Local versus specialist services

HARRY

My pregnancy was normal, until 29 weeks. I started having contractions so my husband took me to our local hospital. I knew it was really early so I was worried, but everyone who examined me kept saying I definitely wasn't going to have the baby today. Despite this, Harry was born just an hour later. The midwife took him from me as he wasn't breathing. He was **intubated** and moved to the **NICU**.

At 24 hours old, Harry had a brain bleed. No one was sure what the outcome of this would be. He could have recovered completely because of his age, or been severely affected. We just didn't know. Harry stayed in hospital for 6 weeks. He was floppy and delayed developmentally. As he got older, we noticed it more. The paediatricians monitored him but didn't know if the delay was linked to his prematurity or the bleed. They told us to 'wait and see'.

After 14 months, Harry was finally diagnosed with **cerebral palsy**. We thought this was coming, but to have a definite diagnosis was so final. Plus, it's hard to explain to people that cerebral palsy isn't one condition but a spectrum.

Family

My family haven't been helpful. My husband describes my dad as 'a character from a Dickens' – it's probably true. Even though they live near us, they've only looked after Harry twice – once was for our wedding anniversary. My husband's mother, on the other hand, gets on with Harry like a house on fire. They can talk for hours and no one else can get a word in edgeways. It's a shame she lives so far away, especially as Harry gets sick on long car journeys.

Ten years after Harry, we had Peter. He's 8 years old now and his relationship with Harry is not always harmonious. He doesn't understand Harry's condition, which he calls 'terrible palsy'. Peter is often impatient with Harry and doesn't like that he gets less time with me because of Harry. It doesn't help that Peter has problems as well: speech delay and **dyspraxia**.

School and Housing

We always wanted Harry to go to the local primary. With this in mind, we negotiated to split his preschool years between the normal preschool, time with a helper and the special school. We wanted Harry to make friends with the children who would then go on to the same primary school as him. Though he has made friends at his school, and now at college, he still finds it easier to talk to adults because of all the one-on-one care he's had.

We managed to get Harry's **statement of educational needs** relatively quickly, mainly because we were prepared early. Other services can be harder to access; for example, one charity which provides assistive equipment. They seemed to be taking a long time to assess Harry so I phoned them. The secretary was very rude and told me to wait. My husband went ballistic at how they treated me and as a result the consultant in charge of assessments called back, being very apologetic and nice. It's not the first time this has happened; we've found that mostly you don't have to fight the person, just the bureaucracy. Individual people are lovely.

Harry's main problems are mobility related. To help him I did **physiotherapy** with him at home and took him for **hydrotherapy** at the local pool. We had to stop the hydrotherapy a few years ago as Harry has got too big to carry into the pool and they don't have a hoist. I stopped the physio recently as well, except during holidays; the college allows him to have three sessions there instead. Harry prefers this – no 17 year old wants to be told to change his posture by his mum.

When Harry was little we could carry him up the stairs to his bedroom, but by 4 years old, neither of us could manage this. We decided to move to a house which had a bedroom downstairs. This was great, especially when Harry started to use a walker. Now he's bigger he has a chair and uses a hoist to get into and out of it. This has meant an expensive redevelopment of the bottom floor of our house. Now it's all open plan and the garden has a raised deck so he can get outside as well.

Holidays

We used to go on holiday. Now it's too hard. First there's the problem of accessibility. Many restaurants and hotels claim they are fully accessible but most are nowhere near. Their idea of accessibility is being able to get in the door – you can forget about going to the toilet.

The other problem is that Harry doesn't like unfamiliar settings. A couple of times we've gone on holiday and had to come back early as Harry just can't handle it. Added to this, Peter has very different ideas of what a holiday means and what he wants to do. The thing is, we don't believe in sending Harry to respite – he should be allowed to stay in his home where he's comfortable and we'll go somewhere. Unfortunately, the system doesn't work like that.

Hospital

Until 2011, all of Harry's medical care was at our local hospital. He has had the same orthopaedic consultant, community paediatrician and physiotherapist for 10 years. We thought this was great until a new surgery was suggested to us. We were due to have a meeting with a new consultant to discuss it, but Harry's orthopaedic consultant talked to him and changed his mind. We began to feel that we needed an independent opinion.

We went to the children's hospital for their opinion. It was just so different from other hospitals. Everyone works as a team, with all the disciplines talking to each other rather than just looking at one section of Harry at a time. Before we had to repeat everything, but not here. The consultants inspire you to feel secure and are only a phone call or email away. We're definitely supporters!

The Future

We have only recently asked for help from the social services – not for us, but to get Harry into the system. He's 18 next year and we're terrified. It means no more children's hospital. We're trying to be hopeful though; our community paediatrician, who we trust completely, has recommended a new orthopaedic surgeon at our local hospital. He treats both adults and children so maybe the transition will be easier....

Journey collected by Rebecca Piper, medical student

GLOSSARY

cerebral palsy: A disorder of movement and posture caused by an insult to the developing brain which can occur before, during or after birth. It can affect children in a number of different ways, including difficulty with movement, communication and swallowing, and varies greatly in severity from very mild to very severe.

dyspraxia: A disorder of physical coordination in which a child can appear as clumsy. They can often be helped by the involvement of an occupational therapist and physiotherapist, who can suggest exercises and aids to help.

hydrotherapy: Special exercises done in warm water.
intubated: Insertion of a breathing tube (endotracheal tube) into the lungs to support breathing.
NICU: Neonatal intensive care unit.
physiotherapy: Helps to provide support with movement when it has been affected by illness, ageing, injury or disability. Specialists in this field are called physiotherapists.
statement of educational needs: A formal document that outlines the needs and the support needed by children who have a condition that affects their ability to learn. This has been replaced by an Education Health Plan.

THEMES FOR DISCUSSION

Information and communication
- Dealing with uncertainty – 'wait and see'

Roles and relationships
- Family dynamics
- Relationships with health professionals

Diagnosis and clinical care
- Impact of a diagnosis such as cerebral palsy and what it means to others

Wider impact of illness
- Social implications of having a chronically unwell child (e.g. for holidays)

Organisation of care and services
- Educational provision for children with special needs
- Transitioning to adult care

HENRY

Well, I guess it's best to start from the beginning. It all started about 5 weeks ago when Henry came home from rugby training with a migraine. He was complaining about his head and said that the sun was hurting his eyes. He just didn't seem himself. It was only when we got home, as he started complaining about a sore throat, that we noticed a lump on his neck. We decided to let Henry take the day off school.

Two days later, Henry went back to school and appeared to be getting better. However, later that day, the school nurse called us to come and pick him up. His migraine had come back, along with the lump on his neck. Henry had never been this ill before, and at this point my wife and I felt it was time to take him to see a doctor. I drove him straight to our local hospital. I remember looking at Henry in the rear view mirror, he seemed in pain and very disorientated. This was the first time I thought that there was something seriously wrong with him.

The doctor in the hospital told us it was most likely a throat infection. He gave Henry some pain killers and reassured us that Henry just needed a few more days to rest and get over his illness. At no point did I doubt the doctor's advice. I mean, how could I challenge his opinion? I work for the council; I don't know anything about all this medical stuff.

Henry did start to get better after that, although I never thought he was back to his normal cheery self. He even managed to go to rugby training the following Saturday. When he got home from training I could tell something was wrong: he didn't want to talk about rugby like he always does. He seemed really drowsy and couldn't say words properly. He was being quite aggressive as well. This all lasted for about 2 hours until he went to sleep. After that, we just couldn't wake him up and then he wet himself. We were so worried at this point and couldn't believe that a throat infection could do this to him. I started to wonder whether he had hit his head at rugby. We rushed him to a different hospital and he was seen straight away by a doctor. Then Henry started to have a **seizure**. We just had to stand there and watch as it all happened. It really is the worst feeling in the world to feel that helpless.

The doctors and nurses couldn't get Henry's seizure under control, so we didn't get much of a chance to talk to them. One of the nurses mentioned that they thought he might have **meningitis**, but they were not sure. I didn't know a lot about that, but I knew it wasn't good. We tried to stay out of the way and let the doctors do their work. Then they came and told us he was being transferred to a specialist hospital. It's funny because we'd both heard of the hospital so I knew he'd be getting the best care possible, but the fact that he was being taken there just made us more worried. They took him to the intensive care unit where he was **ventilated** and then finally transferred him onto the **neurology ward**. After a mad couple of days, we finally got to sit down with the doctors here to talk about Henry.

That brings us to today, so that means we have been here for 5 weeks now. Henry is still having seizures and isn't much better. The doctors are saying he has something called **encephalitis**, but none of the tests have shown exactly what it is. They say it could be autoimmune or viral, but I don't really understand what they mean. I just want to let the doctors do their job so Henry can go home soon.

Every day is a new challenge for us because Henry is so up and down. Since his first seizure, he's been a different person. The hardest thing to get used to has been the change in his behaviour. He has become a very erratic boy. Normally he is like any other teenager, a very shy 13 year old kid, but now he doesn't seem to have any control over what he talks about. It's like he just says the first thing that comes to mind, but half of the stuff he says does not make any sense. I don't think he really understands what has happened to him. He can't concentrate on anything for very long or remember most of his words. His short-term memory is really bad too. He wouldn't be able to remember your name if you came back tomorrow. The most frustrating thing is that Henry will make a little bit of progress, then he'll have another seizure and we're back to square one. It's like being in that movie, you know, *50 First Dates*.

Since we've been here, I have found it really tough. I have never been more worn out in my life. My wife, my sister and I have been rotating who comes and looks after him here. Someone has to be with him all the time because he is so unsteady on his feet. We have three other children, so it's been a real adjustment for us, but we are just trying to make it work. My employers have been really good though; I've used up all my holidays and special leave, but now they just tell me to ring in ill. They have been so understanding and I'm so grateful they are still paying me my wage while this all goes on. My worry is that this cannot go on forever and at some point I will have to leave Henry here and go back to work or risk losing my job.

The lowest point of this all was when we brought the kids in to see Henry. We thought this might help cheer him up because he is constantly asking us when he will be able to go home and he hadn't seen his sisters for 5 weeks. The problem was with our eldest daughter Kate, who is 12. The younger two were just happy to sit and play with him. When Kate saw him, she ran straight out of the room crying. It was as if she didn't recognise Henry as the same person anymore. It has been really tough for her, she keeps asking for her old brother to come back. I thought this would upset Henry, but I guess he isn't really aware of stuff like that at the moment. When Henry does eventually come home, it is going to be a really big adjustment for the girls if things stay like this.

Back home, our family and friends have been such a help. We have a really strong family who have had to deal with disability before. There's a family history of **multiple sclerosis** and a lot of our relatives, like my sister, have been so supportive. They have really helped us cope, and they will do in the future. His friends have also been amazing. His rugby club raised £2000 for him to show their support. That money is going to be so helpful, especially if he is going to need a wheelchair and other help.

In the future, we have a lot of concerns, mainly because the doctors don't know what is wrong with him. There is a lot of frustration for us because we just don't know when we will be able to go home, or at least get transferred back to our local hospital. On the other hand, do we want to rush him out of here to be closer to home – what if the other hospitals aren't as good? After all, Henry was sent here because they couldn't deal with his seizures there. We will just have to deal with whatever happens, but it is really hard when so much is unknown. It is strange because you read about this sort of thing happening in the papers all the time, but you never expect it to be your own kid. It's been a real kick in the teeth.

The best thing about being here has been the nurses. I know it's an amazing facility with the best doctors and technology, but the humour of the nurses makes everything that little bit easier. We have had some really difficult nights where Henry has wet himself, fallen over or had another seizure. When the nurses come to help him they just bring a smile to your face with a little joke. I honestly cannot fault the care we have been given here. You read so much negative stuff in the papers about our hospitals. I just didn't realise how good our health service is.

The doctors think he is going to need a lot of support getting him home and then back into school. They say we may need to adapt our home and that he will need learning aids at school. **Occupational therapy and physiotherapy** both want to help him, while the doctor also mentioned something about **educational psychology**. All of that is just going to be further adjustment for us, but all we want is for Henry to go back to how he was a month ago. Since this happened, it feels like everyone's lives have changed, but you just have to get on with it, don't you?

Journey collected by Samuel Gittens, medical student

GLOSSARY

educational psychology: A branch of psychology that looks at children in an educational environment and at how they learn.

encephalitis: Inflammation of the brain, most commonly caused by a viral infection, which can lead to confusion, seizures and a decreased level of consciousness. It can also, more rarely, be caused by an autoimmune reaction when the body's defence system turns against itself and attacks the body's own cells.

meningitis: Inflammation of the meninges (lining) of the brain and spinal cord, often caused by either a viral or bacterial infection. In older children, it can present with headache, photophobia (dislike of the light), vomiting and fever and requires urgent medical attention.

multiple sclerosis: A neurological condition that can cause a variety of symptoms, including difficulty with tiredness, eyesight, stiff muscles and coordination.

neurology ward: A ward specialising in the care of those with nerve or nervous system problems.

occupational therapy and physiotherapy: Members of the medical multidisciplinary team who work to treat and support patients holistically. Physiotherapists concentrate on physical needs such as helping to clear patients' chests when they have infections or with mobility. Occupational therapists help and support people to be able to complete day-to-day tasks.

seizure: Also known as a *fit*; a seizure is caused by abnormal electrical activity in the brain and can manifest in a number of different ways, including abnormal movements, usually jerking (tonic–clonic seizure), or sometimes stiffness or stillness.

ventilated: When a patient has a tube (endotracheal tube) put down into their lungs and is on a breathing machine called a ventilator to help them breathe.

THEMES FOR DISCUSSION

Information and communication
- Impact of words such as 'meningitis'
- Explaining conditions to family members
- Media depiction of health services

Roles and relationships
- Challenging doctors' decisions
- Supporting role of medical staff

Diagnosis and clinical care
- Behavioural change and psychological diagnoses versus physical diagnoses

Wider impact of illness
- Attitudes and experiences of disability
- Effect on siblings
- 'Taking each day as it comes'

JO

We were travelling down to Cornwall for a holiday after a bad night's sleep because Jo had been up a lot with a cold. We arrived at lunchtime and went to a supermarket to pick up some food and grab a spot of lunch. My wife went and did the shop and I bought lunch for us all in the cafe. I needed a knife and so moved past Jo in the pram, probably pushing her in towards the small table, where she reached up and grabbed a pot of boiling tea and poured it over her leg in the pram. She let out a choking scream which just didn't sound right and you just know you are at a life-defining moment. You can feel the adrenaline kicking in and try to stay calm. It's a bit like keeping your head above water.

My first reactions were good and swift. I took her out of the pram and took her trousers down. Her entire leg came away in my hand and hung down from her ankle, totally freaking out the bystanders, but not me – not at the time. We were in the toilet in a moment and I was looking for cold water. None. The first-aider came over with my wife and eventually an ambulance was called. We waited for a bit, but the sense of panic became unbearable and I decided to drive in my car to the nearest hospital, which wasn't too far away. Action seemed better than inaction.

I drove to the hospital, but when I arrived it all seemed shut down. Eventually and by sheer luck we found the entrance to a working bit of the hospital and the sight of nurses. They started first aid, putting her in cold water, and called a doctor. This was such a relief as you feel you're making poorer and poorer judgements about what is best and you can finally hand over the reins to professionals who know what to do. The ambulance eventually caught up with us and took us to the nearest general hospital, and from there to the specialist burns unit some 4 or 5 hours later.

The ambulance staff were great. They are a different breed – able to span both worlds. The medics at the general hospital were less than decisive, not giving some drugs because they didn't know how much to give to one of Jo's age. We had calmed considerably by then and my wife had to force them to call the paediatrics department to get advice on this matter. You realise you do have to take responsibility.

The burns unit was full of excellent folk dedicated to the sort of knowledge we desperately needed. But the news just kept getting worse and worse. Every doctor that walked in had some bad news and a range of options that was explained, and the next time they came in with a test result in their hand, the very worst of those options had happened. This occurred time and time again. We were looking at a doctor's face when they walked in a room to see what they were thinking. Gradually, things became graver and graver. We felt like Jo was slipping away from us. Finally, things came to a head as Jo showed signs of going into **toxic shock**. We knew by this time what this meant and how serious her situation was. A day before we had a perfect child; then we were told she would be scarred for life; now though, we would be lucky to walk out with her alive. It really is quite a journey to take in little more than a weekend.

At each stage we were told as much as we wanted. The explanations were clear. If we had a question it was always answered. At this point, you feel you are trying to read into the mind of the medic. What do they really mean? Because they have to be diplomatic and never raise hopes, but never point out the worst, and burns are difficult to understand. How will my child look in 5 years, 10 years? They don't know – the range is so large. It's difficult to predict outcomes, and that adds to the sense of uncertainty. But we knew Jo's was a very bad burn indeed.

We ended up in the city hospital for 2 weeks where Jo went through several operations. During this time, I recall being approached by someone who was clearly asking about how it happened with a view to child protection. I didn't mind then – and I don't mind to this day, but I wonder if everyone would take that view in our position – after all, this was an accident that happened in a public supermarket at midday.

Jo was transferred to our local burns unit. It's a difficult place to get to, but the staff are good and we have regular check-ups. Jo had the best part of a year in a compression garment which never seemed to fit correctly – and needed massaging and **Kelo-cote** applied on a daily basis, which for a girl in nappies was time consuming – particularly with her younger sister in the background.

Jo is nearly 3 now. She is a very lively and active child with an enquiring mind. She hasn't asked about her leg and it is looking amazingly good. It really seems to have done well over the last year. I guess we will have to deal with questions when they come. It might be good to get some advice about that.

Journey collected by Chloe Macaulay, Paediatrician

GLOSSARY

Kelo-cote: A dressing used for burns.

toxic shock syndrome: A serious, potentially fatal condition caused by the release of bacterial toxins into the bloodstream. It can cause a temperature and rash, diarrhoea and low blood pressure.

THEMES FOR DISCUSSION

Information and communication
- Use of words

Roles and relationships
- Parental roles

Diagnosis and clinical care
- Safeguarding procedures

Wider impact of illness
- Reactions to accidents/life-changing events

Organisation of care and services
- Organisation of emergency services and departments
- Local versus specialist units
- Visiting and sleeping arrangements for families

KATY

Katy, our second of four children, was born by caesarean section. Once we were discharged, I took her for her neonatal hearing test, which she failed. I had gone on my own and could see the doctors' grave reactions as they looked at the results on a screen (the consultation room had a glass window so I could see through to where they were). I was not surprised therefore when they came through and told me the results. At the time, I thought, well, at least she's just deaf – we can cope with that I think…

Katy hit no real milestones on time. She was late sitting up; she didn't gurgle or make sounds apart from a strange screaming noise; she struggled to crawl. My mother-in-law noticed her development seemed slow and urged us to get her referred to the community health visitor. The health visitor assured us that nothing was wrong but said she could refer us to our local child development centre if we really wanted to.

Katy was then seen by a succession of paediatricians who offered no real advice and relied almost entirely on our observations rather than on any detailed investigations of Katy herself and we made little headway there. We were also unhappy with the audiology service locally and, using private health insurance, asked for Katy to be referred to a consultant **audiologist**. We duly saw a consultant who conducted a number of tests that confirmed Katy's diagnosis of moderate **sensorineural hearing loss**. He subsequently referred Katy to a children's hospital for further genetic investigation to determine the underlying causes of Katy's deafness. On top of this, we were referred to the **neurologist** and she was diagnosed in their clinic when she was two and a half with **Moebius syndrome**.

Katy never ate well and, on the advice of a dietician, we continued to build up her tolerance to solid/lumpy food, but then she had a choking episode, which was extremely scary. After this, we demanded that her swallowing be reviewed, so she was referred for a **videofluoroscopy**. This showed she had significant delays in swallowing and the recommendation was that she only eat pureed food. It was becoming a huge strain to maintain her food and fluid intake at necessary levels and this began to dominate all aspects of family mealtimes.

Katy began to fall a lot, so we asked that she be assessed again by the paediatrician, who recommended a helmet. At this stage, Katy was also fitted with a second skin (Lycra suit) to give her more stability, as she was beginning to show a curvature of the spine, and for a limited time this helped with her posture. We began to get more concerned about her developmental delay and she was referred to a specialist child development centre. Katy has very limited speech and shows autistic tendencies. She was assessed as being on the autistic spectrum, albeit at the low end.

We attended a conference in the States run by the US Moebius Foundation. We then started to challenge the initial diagnosis and started pushing for her specialists to take another look. Given her muscle deterioration, we were referred to two **orthopaedic** consultants to examine her deteriorating legs and her spine. She was diagnosed with **hyperlordosis** of the spine and ended up with a brace which fits round her abdomen, which she still wears today. It was about this time that we had to try and choose a school for Katy.

In April 2009, I went on maternity leave for the fourth time (we had decided to have another child again on the advice that any child would have a very low risk of inheriting Moebius). By June 2009, we and the school had noticed Katy's walking deteriorating significantly. By then she had a walker, but seemed to be able to use it less and less effectively. I asked at the school therapist meeting for a referral by the local paediatrician to see a muscle doctor to review her legs and spine again.

I had a new baby to cope with and numerous medical specialists for Katy with no clear path of what the next steps were. Around that time, we also decided that Katy should have a **gastrostomy** tube, which has really helped her thrive.

In November 2009, we went to see the neuromuscular consultants at the children's hospital. We were there all day and at the end were told that they were fairly sure Katy had in fact got **FSH**, that she was in the 10% severe category and that she would be in a wheelchair. We listened and said it was what we had expected following the deterioration in her walking, but the next 2 or 3 weeks were a blur. They also examined me as they thought I showed signs of the condition.

The results took an incredibly long time to come through, and in April 2010, we were called back to get the results. This time we knew it would be confirmed, but it still came as a shock to see the results written down on paper. It is also clear with this condition that there is no real hope of physical improvement – just a gradual deterioration. At the same appointment, they mentioned that I should see the adult neuromuscular consultants and referred me for assessment. They touched on the possibility that I could be a carrier. They also said it could affect our other children.

At the end of June 2009, Katy went into a wheelchair. Katy has also met the criteria of our local hospice as having a life-limiting condition.

It is a wholly traumatic journey to be faced with and one which we were not expecting. In sum, the last 6 years would have been better and less stressful if there had been coordination between the multi-agency care which Katy has needed – NHS, social services, therapists and education. We have had to chase a number of doctors who told us that they would refer Katy to other doctors – patients are anxious to receive these referrals and do not want to wait months before they even receive a copy of the referral letter.

At its peak, we have three or four appointments per week at different hospitals and community trusts. There is a lot of juggling and the need to rearrange appointments, etc. All that being said, we are immensely grateful for the help we have received over the years from the medical profession, which is packed full of caring and dedicated people.

The strain on the siblings is hard to measure now, but is something that we are constantly aware of. Our wider families have also been a support, but privately have no doubt struggled with what we are going through. We cannot look ahead – we are living for the moment as it is too difficult to comprehend the reality of what we have now and what we will face in the future. Despite this, Katy is a delightful, funny and caring child and forms an integral part of our family.

Journey written by Katy's mother

GLOSSARY

audiologist: A professional who specialises in hearing.

FSH: Facioscapulohumeral muscular dystrophy – a form of muscular dystrophy characterised by loss of muscle strength, in particular in the face, back and upper arms, but it may affect other areas too. It varies in severity and associated features, but can include deafness and lordosis. It is progressive – getting worse over time – and can be dominantly inherited (www.fshsociety.org).

gastrostomy: A small tube inserted through the skin of the abdominal wall and into the stomach in order to administer nutrition and medicines directly into the stomach (also known as a PEG or percutaneous endoscopic gastrostomy). It is inserted in an operating theatre while the child is under general anesthetic.

hyperlordosis: An excessive curvature of the spine.
Moebius syndrome: A rare neurological disorder characterised by weak
     facial muscles and other physical abnormalities.
neurologist: A doctor who specialises in the study of the nervous system.
orthopaedic: Specialising in the musculoskeletal system.
sensorineural hearing loss: A type of deafness that occurs when there is
     damage to the inner ear or the nerve pathways between the inner
     ear and the brain. It can be mild, moderate or severe.
videofluoroscopy: A type of X-ray test to assess swallowing.

THEMES FOR DISCUSSION

Information and communication
- Non-verbal communication
- Communication between teams

Roles and relationships
- 'Expert parents'
- Team working
- Support for families

Diagnosis and clinical care
- Uncertainty

Wider impact of illness
- Impact on family life

Organisation of care and services
- Coordination between teams and services

LAURA

I've got a history of complications with my pregnancies. On my first baby's 3-month scan, they picked up a high **nuchal translucency**, so we went through lots of tests which all looked fine. At 33 weeks and 2 days, I stopped feeling the baby moving, so I called my midwife and she told me to go to the hospital. They monitored everything; he still had a heartbeat but the trace wasn't great, so they decided to deliver. When he was delivered we didn't hear him cry. He had **hydrops foetalis** affecting his lungs, so his heart was beating but he couldn't breathe. They tried to resuscitate him for 20 minutes, they did everything they could, but it just wasn't successful. We named him Jack.

There was definitely something genetic going on because he had something wrong with his lungs, his kidneys and – I couldn't see anything wrong with his face or features, but they know what they're looking for – they said his ears were a certain shape. They told us as much as they could, but they haven't been able to identify a specific cause or syndrome. Recently, I've been in touch with a geneticist, and there's a study going on. They'll test Jack's blood (preserved from autopsy) and mine and my husband's saliva, so maybe in the next year or so we might find out. I would like to find out for my children's future, you know, I would just like to know.

We got pregnant again with my son, Peter, who is about to turn 3. I had lots of appointments. The biggest check-up for us was the 3-month scan because that's where they first noticed a problem last time. Then I started getting headaches. On the morning Peter was born I had a **seizure**. It was **pre-eclampsia**, but there had been no other warning signs. At the last midwife appointment, she mentioned that my blood pressure was slightly elevated, but I didn't know much about pre-eclampsia, and she didn't seem too concerned. The seizures were quite scary on reflection. For a long time I had anxiety about them because you can continue to have seizures after you deliver. Even now, I check my blood pressure every day. If ever I have a headache or a funny feeling I just panic, thinking that I'm going to have a seizure. I think it's going to haunt me for a while.

We decided we would have another baby after Peter, even though it was a risk considering all the previous complications. We met with the consultant, and he said the risk was more about what happened with Jack than the pre-eclampsia, even though the pre-eclampsia was probably what scared us the most... because what if something happened to me? I have my son to think about as well.

The 3-month scan was absolutely fine. I had been monitoring my blood pressure and protein every day, having lots of midwife appointments and outpatient appointments; everything was perfect.

Two days before Christmas (I was 29 weeks pregnant), I went for a routine scan, which showed I had **polyhydramnios**. The doctor explained that it could be nothing, some women just have more fluid, but in a lot of cases it means that there's something more sinister going on. He said it could be a blockage of the oesophagus (**oesophageal atresia**), but they couldn't be sure, so he referred us right away. We were seen the next day, Christmas Eve.

They offered us an **amniocentesis**, but explained that it could prompt early labour. We would only do an amniocentesis to find out if there was something wrong, and then act upon it; in other words, whether to terminate the pregnancy. We decided that we weren't going to take the risk. We were going to continue with the pregnancy no matter what.

We went for another scan around 6th January, by which point I was really uncomfortable. The consultant said I needed a drainage, which happened the next day, but at my next scan the fluid had gone up again. We were still hoping they would say everything was fine, as it was still a possibility. Everything seemed fine, she was growing, her heartbeat was OK, so there were a lot of positives.

We were told that if my waters broke or if I had any contractions, I should go straight to the local hospital, and that we shouldn't try to get into central London. That scared us slightly, thinking, is our local going to be equipped in the same way that the specialist hospital would be?

At about 00:45, I woke up and my waters had broken. We had rehearsed everything so much, and it was good that we had, as we both knew exactly what to do. My midwife had written on my notes what Charlie, my husband, would need to say to the ambulance. I had written everything on the birth plan. It said, 'I have to have a C-section, this is what I need you to do', and in red, 'First child: hydrops, second child: pre-eclampsia, this pregnancy: polyhydramnios'. I had to shout to Charlie some of the things to say, he did really well, but I think he panicked!

I've had a caesarean section three times but this was by far the most urgent. With the others there was time to talk about things beforehand. The baby's heartbeat dropped to 60, so they said they needed to do a **general anaesthetic**. They told Charlie that he couldn't come in, and I was panicking, thinking, 'Oh my God, what's happening?'

We were still hoping she would be fine. Initially, someone told us that everything was OK, and we were thinking 'fantastic', but when the doctors came back they told us that she did have the oesophageal atresia. They said that she'd had some breathing difficulties so they'd given her oxygen, but only a small amount, she was breathing OK for herself… she just needed a little help.

Because of the caesarean, I couldn't go to see her, but they brought her round to me when she was ready to be transferred. It was just for a minute, and that was difficult, not being able to spend time with her, but I was really grateful to see her at all. She was in an **incubator** and she was all covered up, I touched her toes and she wiggled them, which was nice. The next time I saw her was 3 days later.

Initially, all we were expecting was the atresia. The consultant said that, unless there were any other underlying issues, then she could be a normal healthy child and grow to adulthood just fine. She might need multiple surgeries and have problems with swallowing and eating, and there will be lots of people involved in her care, but, you know, the outlook is good.

Since we've been here (at the children's hospital), however, the news has changed. They have operated on the atresia, and she seems to be doing great in terms of recovering. They've also noticed that she has a blockage in her nose, so they need to operate again – they're planning to do that on Monday. Initially, they detected one hole in the heart, but now they have detected another, so that will mean further surgery. I'm hoping that they'll do this nose surgery and then she'll be able to come home, and the heart surgery will happen later. Of course, it's whatever's best for her, but I just want her home as soon as possible.

Because there are multiple problems, they think there is something underlying; they think she could have **CHARGE syndrome**. I hadn't heard of it until now and I've read up a little about it, trying not to scare myself. Some of the signs can't be picked up until she's developing and growing. They can do a test for it, but even if it's negative, it isn't 100% guaranteed to be correct.

Initially, we were told that we were looking at about 3 weeks here, but when we spoke to the consultant yesterday, he said that it could be a couple of months. If that's the case, Charlie and I will be ships passing in the night. Each one of us will spend half the week here and then half with Peter at home. It's going to be a major upheaval for him not having us both there, but it's the next best thing.

Throughout the pregnancy, my son has been OK. I mean, obviously children play up, but in general he has been absolutely fine, and really excited. When I came home, his first question was 'where's my baby?' and he was asking about this for a day or two, but then he lost a bit of interest. Yesterday he got upset, and his teacher said that he was crying and asking for me. Everyone keeps saying that he'll be fine, but it does have... sorry ... if it was just me and Charlie having to deal with this it would be fine, but I keep thinking about the impact it's going to have on him.

Our friends and family have been amazing, but they were always trying to reassure us – I suppose that's natural. It doesn't reassure me, nobody can give me any guarantees. They tried to reassure me the first time and I lost a child. That's something that my husband and I have to battle with, individually, and as a couple. Nobody else can really understand that. My biggest blessing is that whatever we go through now, at least she's here, and she's doing well.

We've got a lot to deal with at the moment, and we're just thinking in terms of what that means for her, her future and our family. We can only process it day by day. What I've found is that it's normally when everything stops that it hits you.

Journey collected by Sabie Rainton, medical student

GLOSSARY

amniocentesis: A test that can be performed when a woman is pregnant to look for chromosomal conditions (such as Down syndrome) or infection in the foetus. It involves a needle being inserted through the abdomen and into the amniotic sac surrounding the foetus to remove some amniotic fluid. This fluid contains foetal cells which can then be analysed.

CHARGE syndrome: A genetic condition characterised by the presence of a number of unusual features. CHARGE stands for
- Coloboma (a defect of the eye)
- Heart defects
- Atresia choanae (narrowing of or blind-ending nostrils)
- Retardation of growth and development
- Genital abnormalities
- Ear abnormalities

general anaesthetic: A drug that has the ability to bring about a reversible loss of consciousness. Anaesthetists administer these drugs to induce or maintain general anaesthesia to facilitate surgery.

hydrops foetalis: Where there is an accumulation of excess fluid in two or more areas of a foetus or new-born baby, such as the lungs, heart or abdomen. It is often serious and is the result of an underlying condition such as rhesus disease, severe anaemia, heart or lung failure or an underlying genetic disorder.

incubator: A clear plastic apparatus that provides a controlled environment for a baby (e.g. warmth, humidity and oxygen if needed).

nuchal translucency: A text performed on women when they are 11–14 weeks pregnant that estimates the chance that the baby has a chromosomal disorder. The fluid at the back of the foetus's neck is measured by ultrasound scan, and an increased thickness can be indicative of an underlying chromosomal disorder such as Down syndrome.

oesophageal atresia: When the oesophagus (or feeding tube) is blind-ending (i.e. it starts at the mouth but does not join the stomach as normal). Babies with oesophageal atresia require potentially complicated surgery to correct the condition. It can present antenatally (before birth) with polyhydramnios.

polyhydramnios: Excessive fluid is noted to be surrounding the foetus on an antenatal ultrasound scan. Often the cause is unknown, but it can be associated with illness in the mother, including maternal heart disease or diabetes. Rarely, it can be an indication that the baby is not able to swallow properly due to a problem with its gastrointestinal tract.

pre-eclampsia: A condition that can occur in pregnancy, causing a woman to develop high blood pressure, protein in her urine and sometimes swollen feet. It needs to be monitored and treated carefully, in some cases by delivering the baby, as the complications can be dangerous to both mother and baby. A rare but serious complication is the development of eclampsia, which causes seizures in the mother and can be life threatening.

seizure: Also known as a *fit*; a seizure is caused by abnormal electrical activity in the brain and can manifest in a number of different ways, including abnormal movements, usually jerking or sometimes stiffness or stillness.

THEMES FOR DISCUSSION

Information and communication
- Reading up on conditions and sources of information

Roles and relationships
- Trust in medical profession

Diagnosis and clinical care
- The need to separate babies from their mothers after caesarean section if babies need to go to neonatal intensive care

Wider impact of illness
- Impact of a stillbirth
- Impact of death and illness on families, siblings and marital relationships

Organisation of care and services
- Autopsies for stillbirths
- Tertiary (level 3) neonatal units versus local (levels 1–2) neonatal units

LILY

When Lily was two and a half years old, she started feeling very tired. She would be flat out on the sofa and nothing would make her feel better. We took her to see the GP, but were told that there was nothing wrong. Her gums then started bleeding and she was getting a lot of bruises. We took her back to the GP and then to A&E that same month, but were again told that she was fine. We knew that something was not right as she had never been a sick child. She didn't get colds and she was never ill. We took her to A&E again, and luckily the doctor who saw her had done **oncology**. She recognised her symptoms and knew straightaway what was wrong. She was diagnosed with **acute myeloid leukaemia**. It was just a simple blood test that was needed to diagnose her, but no one had thought to do it before.

She then started **chemotherapy**. After her first round, the doctors noticed that she had a distended tummy. They thought that her bowels had ruptured, and took her to theatre to investigate because they couldn't see much on the X-ray. When she was given the **general anaesthetic**, she had a cardiac arrest. It lasted 8 minutes. The doctors managed to stabilise her and the operation was stopped. She was **ventilated** for 3 weeks in the **PICU**; she was unstable and on a lot of drugs. It was then that Lily was diagnosed with **dilated cardiomyopathy**, which happened as a result of her chemotherapy, and that the doctors first mentioned that she would need a heart transplant. There is only a 5% chance of children getting dilated cardiomyopathy following chemotherapy, so it wasn't the first thing that the doctors thought was happening. We were dealing with one problem and then suddenly it became many other problems – it was horrible.

The heart transplant was not a route that Lily could go down immediately because her leukaemia treatment had not finished. The doctors didn't want her to stop chemotherapy as there was a high chance that the leukaemia could come back. She managed to finish her chemotherapy about a year later and she was stable on heart medication for another 6 months. She then deteriorated rapidly. The doctors increased her heart medication as much as they could, but it was not helping. She was admitted to hospital on **milrinone** for 3 months while we waited for a bed to become available at the specialist centre.

We had hoped that she would be listed for transplantation then, but while we were at the specialist centre, she had a study to measure her blood pressure. We found out that the pressure in her lungs was much higher than expected. This was yet another setback for Lily, as it stopped her again from being listed for transplantation. The doctors didn't know what to do. They sent her home on **sildenafil** to get the pressure down, but they didn't think that it would work. She had been in situations like this before so we were positive that she would turn it around. We never lost hope. She didn't fail this time. We went back for another study 3 months later, and the pressure in her lungs had gone down significantly, so she was finally able to be listed for a heart transplant.

She then went through a period when the medication stopped working – she was growing bigger and her heart wasn't coping. The doctors suggested putting Lily on the **Berlin heart** while she waited for her heart transplant. It was nice to have an option when before we didn't have any. But then Lily started doing really well again – she was enjoying herself and was like a normal 5 year old. We didn't want to take her to hospital while she was doing well, but we also didn't want her to get so unwell so that she didn't have that option at all – it was a very fine balance. A few weeks later, she caught a cold and went downhill really quickly. The decision for her to have the Berlin heart was taken out of our hands.

The last time we were at the centre, Lily became close friends with a girl who had a Berlin heart, so we knew what to expect. She very quickly got used to being attached to the machine, having a big dressing and only being able to go to certain places. She felt much better on the Berlin heart and I think that she understood that it was helping her so she wasn't bothered by it – it was quite amazing! Being in hospital for 5 months on the Berlin heart allowed Lily to do things that she would not have been able to do had she been at home as she was feeling so well. Had we been at home, she would have probably been in and out of hospital many times, considering how poorly she had been before.

I stay with Lily every day while she is in hospital. We live 40 miles away so I have been living with my younger daughter, Sophie, in accommodation nearby provided by a charity. Having Sophie with us in hospital was easy initially because she was only 5 months old and she wasn't doing much. I could entertain her just with a book or a toy. She is now 10 months old so it is harder work, but she has kept me occupied, so time has gone by really quickly. It has been nice to have a good distraction and it has been good for Lily to have someone else around too. If I just had Lily, I would have probably spent a lot of time sitting around and thinking about things.

It seems strange to say that being in hospital has not been that bad because Lily has been really well and she has been able to do a lot of things. She has made many friends, gone to Pizza Express and has even met the band One Direction! She has also been going to school here, which she really enjoys; she wasn't even going to school before because she was too ill. The teachers come up to her because she is on **immunosuppressants** and cannot be around other children at the moment. She really loves cooking. The school gets a chef to come in from different places – yesterday one came from Buckingham Palace! The volunteers who come to the ward are really helpful too. The same ones come every week on the same day so you get used to seeing them around.

Lily had her heart transplant 2 weeks ago. You know that you are waiting for it and that it is going to happen sometime, but you never think that it will be today. We had a couple of false alarms before, so we had a lot of practice. When we received the phone call, we didn't get our hopes up. Everything happened so quickly compared to the other times. Lily had just woken up so she didn't have much time to think about it, but she was very calm and excited that she would be able to go home and do many things. She sailed through the transplant and everything else since.

When we were told that Lily had leukaemia, it was horrible because we had never been in a medical situation before. But as time goes on, you get tougher and tougher. One problem becomes many others, but you deal with them. The transplant had been in the pipeline for nearly 3 years so we were mentally prepared, but there were always things stopping her from having it. There were times when we thought that she would never have one, but she is a fighter and she has made it. Lily is being discharged today and we are looking forward to finally going home with a brighter future in sight.

Journey collected by Sara Tho-Calvi, medical student

GLOSSARY

acute myeloid leukaemia (AML): A form of cancer of the blood which affects the myeloid line of white cells. It often presents with bleeding, particularly from the gums, and bruising, as well as being pale and tired. AML requires aggressive treatment with chemotherapy and can be life threatening.

Berlin heart: A pump that sits outside the body and takes over the work of a patient's heart when it is too weak to pump blood around the body itself. It is often used as a holding measure while waiting for a heart transplant.

chemotherapy: A range of chemical substances that act in different ways to kill cancer cells. They all have side effects which may include hair loss, increased susceptibility to infections and damage to other organs, such as the heart or lungs.

dilated cardiomyopathy: A condition in which the muscle of the heart becomes weak and baggy and is unable to function properly, often leading to heart failure. There are a number of different causes; for example, one can be born with it or it can develop secondary to a viral infection or sometimes secondary to other problems in the heart.

general anaesthetic: A drug that has the ability to bring about a reversible loss of consciousness. Anaesthetists administer these drugs to induce or maintain general anaesthesia to facilitate surgery.

immunosuppressants: Drugs that suppress the body's natural immune system (defence system). Immunosuppression can be intentional, such as in the case of a transplant, where it is used to prevent the body attacking the newly transplanted organ. It can also be a side effect of some drugs, such as the chemotherapy agents used for cancer.

milrinone: A medication given through the veins to help patients in heart failure.

oncology: The study of cancer.

PICU: Paediatric intensive care unit.

sildenafil: A medication given to help reduce excessive pressure in the blood vessels going through the lungs (called pulmonary hypertension).

ventilated: When a patient has a tube put down into their lungs and is on a breathing machine called a ventilator to help them breathe.

THEMES FOR DISCUSSION

Information and communication
- Understanding the risks and benefits of treatment

Roles and relationships
- Medicalisation of families and the expert parent

Diagnosis and clinical care
- Rare conditions
- Intensive care settings

Wider impact of illness
- How families adapt
- Effect on siblings

Organisation of care and services
- Schooling for ill children

LUKE

One shuttlecock went up but two came down. I initially passed the double vision off as nothing; I was not prepared to wear glasses at the age of 17. However, when I suddenly started to vomit, develop severe headaches and had difficulties in falling asleep, my mother forced me to visit the GP. I knew this was serious when he referred me to the consultant **neurologist** at my local hospital. Within the space of a week, I had several brain scans and multiple blood tests. The doctor saw a lump on day six and I was then whisked off to the **oncology team** at another hospital that night. No warning or explanation, just the word 'oncology'.

Three days later the hospital arranged for my parents to meet the consultant who was in charge of my treatment. They knew it was bad news when they walked into the room and saw a large crowd of doctors observing my brains scans. The consultant sat them down and explained that there was no time to waste. **Chemotherapy** had to start immediately. I was told that I had a 'rapidly progressing, **malignant pineal parenchymal tumour**' and that there was 'about a 47% 5-year survival rate'. This arbitrary figure was what my parents took away from that consultation. No other information seemed to make any impression on them after hearing this.

My memories of the first week of treatment are all distorted. All I can remember is drifting in and out of consciousness. I was not aware of where I was, or what was being done to me. My mother made all the treatment decisions for me because I was in no state to do so myself. When I was awake, I was either fighting back the urge to vomit or I was numb from all the painkillers I was given. Mum still wanted the chemotherapy to go ahead.

It was only after the first week of treatment had ended that I realised I was being treated for cancer. Until that point, I was too exhausted to even contemplate my diagnosis. I figured that you only ever hear these stories on the radio or read about them in the newspaper. You never imagine that it could affect you. When it does, you quickly learn what matters – to me, it was my family and my wellbeing. A few weeks ago, I was a happy and healthy young man, and just like that, everything became insignificant. It finally struck me that I was fighting for my life.

It was difficult for my mother to accept the diagnosis. She was very emotional and just could not understand why this had happened to her. Even now, she hates to talk about my year in hospital. It was as if her perfect little boy had been consumed by this illness, and the result was someone who 'was not her son'.

My father, however, was the complete opposite; he did a lot of research around the cancer. He spoke to the doctors and borrowed books which helped him to learn all about why the tumour arises and what the future may hold. He knew exactly what medications I was given and all their side effects. This helped him to cope. It gave him a purpose, something to occupy him during the day whilst I was knocked out from the chemotherapy. He became an expert in my condition so that he could help fight my battles for me.

I was allowed a home visit every weekend during my therapy. During the second weekend at home, I developed an infection and my parents rushed me to the local emergency department. We had to wait for over 7 hours just to access a bed and to see a doctor. I was in agony and all I remember is the endless wait. There was no way to monitor my condition in the waiting room. I felt so vulnerable there. I was dependent on others to take care of my every need. I hated being stripped of my independence, but I was in excruciating pain so I had no choice. I simply could not move and I really thought that that was it for me. I told my father to 'kill me now'. It was the first time during the course of my illness that I had seen my father cry. In retrospect, I wish that the hospital had done something to alleviate my pain and make me feel comfortable whilst we were waiting for a bed. Perhaps I would have been able to cope better and would have saved my father from having to hear that.

Do I regret asking my father to kill me? Of course I do, but mostly because of the effect it had on my younger sister, Renee. I realise that no one actually took the time to explain to her what was going on. There was never time for my parents to look after Renee. The focus was always on me – I became the world that they revolved around and Renee was forced to grow up in my shadow.

During my time in hospital, Renee had become withdrawn at school and she hardly spoke when she came to visit. This was very unlike her normal, bubbly self. I wish that I had taken the opportunity myself to explain the condition to her. She was only 7; there was no way she would have understood what was going on. At that age, she would have craved stability and safety, and no one was there to provide this for her. My parents barely had the time to speak to each other, and when they did, it was always about me: an update on my feeding and weight status or the latest information about my treatment. When they were not at the hospital, my father was at work or my mother struggled to pay the bills. Renee's personal and educational needs were the least of their priorities at the time. I still feel guilty for stealing away her childhood. I didn't mind my disease killing me, but it hurt because it was killing my family too.

The chemotherapy seemed to be working well over the next few weeks, or so I believed. I remember feeling a sense of overwhelming relief every time I completed a block of chemotherapy and I was allowed to go back home. I just kept thinking, 'I am now one step closer to finishing treatment', and this kept me motivated.

However, this newfound hope did not last very long. Three months into my treatment, I started developing severe back pains. Every time I changed position on the bed, I felt a searing pain shoot down my spine. On the numerous occasions when I told my consultant that I was suffering from back pain, he simply reassured me that 'all would be fine'. Although this was meant to be comforting, I still felt uneasy hearing this. It made me question whether I was fabricating the pain. My parents were extremely worried and they fought hard for his attention. However, we were initially told that it was 'just the side effects of chemotherapy' – my parents knew something was not right though. The consultant never took notice of me, prescribing me useless painkillers that did nothing. At the same time, my mother realised that my mobility was deteriorating rapidly. I felt like I was falling apart.

Two months after the back pains started, I finally managed to get some of the answers I wanted when the consultant and his team came into my room to discuss the plan for **radiotherapy**. The oncology team had already spoken to my parents without me knowing, but it was my turn now. He told me that they were planning to irradiate my back because there were several **metastatic tumours** down my spine. That was the reason for my back pains. He did not want to tell me earlier because he felt I was not in the right state of mind to be able to process and cope with such news. He felt that I already had enough to deal with, let alone know that the chemotherapy was not being as effective as they had anticipated.

My mother was always adamant that I was to be told of the situation because she understood how I liked to be in as much control as possible over my condition. My father was impartial. He hated to be the bearer of bad news and just could not contemplate telling me this. It would have been too distressing. He always found it hard to see me upset. I feel as though hiding this new diagnosis from me made it seem 'less real' for my father – it was almost a form of denial.

When people ask me if I am angry at the doctors for withholding this information from me, I reply 'no'. I suppose they were trying to protect me from further distress. They were only acting according to my best interests at the time. It gave me hope to hear them say it would all be OK in the end. It gave me something to cling onto, even if in the end, it was all just a false pretence.

Thirty-five radiotherapy sessions and a year later, I am now in **remission**. People don't realise the transition into recovery is a challenge in itself. I have lost my friends and my independence along the way. I look in the mirror and I see a young boy, still without any hair; it is a constant reminder that cancer has moulded me into someone different. Being part of the Teenage Cancer Centre throughout my treatment really helped me to conquer my personal demons that threatened to bring me down when I was hurting from chemotherapy or struggling with radiotherapy. It allowed me to meet others who were going through the same ordeal and this gave me hope to continue fighting.

I was told that I may only have a few years left to live. What's the point of having a timer on your life though? It only prevents you from living. I want to enjoy every day I have with my friends and family. I am uncertain of how long I have left, but the way I see it is that I am blessed to have won my life back.

Journey collected by Karishma Desai, medical student

GLOSSARY

chemotherapy: A number of drugs that are used for the treatment of cancer. There are a wide variety of different types of chemotherapy which target cancerous cells in different ways. All have side effects which vary dependent on the type of drug, but may include hair loss, nausea and vomiting.

malignant pineal parenchymal tumour: A type of cancer originating from the pineal gland in the brain. The most common presenting symptoms are headache, nausea and vomiting.

metastatic tumours: Tumours that develop secondary to a 'primary' tumour elsewhere. Different types of cancer metastasise to different areas; for example, many types of brain tumour may metastasise to the spine.

neurologist: A doctor who specialises in nerves and the nervous system.

oncology team: A team of professionals specialising in cancer care.

radiotherapy: A treatment combination used for certain types of cancer which involves firing beams of high-energy radiation ('irradiation') at the tumour. Side effects are common and include soreness of the skin and damage to the areas adjacent to the tumour.

remission: Can be complete or partial. Complete remission refers to the state in which there is no identifiable cancer in the body following treatment, whereas partial remission indicates that the cancer has reduced or has stopped growing.

THEMES FOR DISCUSSION

Information and communication
- Impact of words such as 'oncology', and statistics
- How much information to give

Roles and relationships
- Autonomy and consent in young people/adolescence
- Having a sibling with cancer
- The 'expert patient'
- Paternalism

Diagnosis and clinical care
- Long term effects of cancer treatments

Wider impact of illness
- Physical stigmata of certain conditions; for example, losing your hair
- Being a teenager with a long term condition (LTC)

Organisation of care and services
- Financial support available for families with children with LTCs

MIKEY

When Mikey was about 15 months old, he first started showing signs of being very thirsty and weeing large amounts. We would put him to bed with several nappies on. About 2 months later, we had a babysitter who said that there was something odd about him. He had got up twice. He couldn't say 'mummy' or 'daddy' yet, but he could say the word for water. At that point, it clicked that he was **diabetic**. I am a diabetic so I knew the signs.

It took us another 2 days to do a test because I was so horrified that my baby was diabetic. I phoned the local GP and she said to come in and pick up a letter and then take him to the local hospital. I said no, you fax a letter to the hospital and we'll go straight there, which we did. At the hospital, I had to deal with the shock that my tiny baby had diabetes, even though I knew about it. I remember being in a very hot ward in the middle of August and we were in for a week. At that time, Mikey's brother was three and a half.

Mikey is a showman so any attention he would get was terrific, but my experience was not as positive. I got the feeling that the team weren't experienced in dealing with a child of his age with diabetes. They didn't give me answers. The consultant referred to another consultant at another hospital, which I found very frustrating.

The diabetic nurse specialist said to me, 'You know all about diabetes, here's the pen, give him an injection'. She used terrible wording: 'If you get the blood sugars too low you'll damage his brain, if you get them too high you'll damage his organs and body'. We were there with a baby whose sugars were fluctuating all over the place. I was in a total panic. We didn't know at any point if Mikey was **hypo** or **hyper**.

All our attention went to Mikey and I became very short fused and angry with the older one, who I felt should just get on with things. He was going to nursery and would cry and cry.

I was having weekly phone calls from the nurse, but she wasn't helping me with the questions I had. She would say things that really should have been said in a much better way and would send me into a panic. I was stressed out like that for a year and a half until we started looking for a new consultant and we changed hospitals to the person who our first consultant had always been consulting. That has been an incredibly positive move. He's on the ball. He knows the answers. I get it from him direct. The team is great. Mikey's still fairly unstable, but is very active and they help take control of his diabetes.

When we first wanted to send Mikey to nursery, we couldn't find anywhere that would take him. Luckily, I have a friend who is a psychologist and she mentioned that there was some money available locally for children who otherwise couldn't access education. Within 2 months, the council had found a pot of money which meant that Mikey could have a full-time carer in a nursery. We were able to interview the person who would be his carer, although it took about 2 years for us to actually get the money for him.

He has a watch that beeps and tells him when he has to do a blood test in school – four times a day. He has a wheel that tells him how much **insulin** to give depending on what the blood sugar is.

Mikey has collapsed once and I called 999. He was hypo. He hasn't had any acute admissions though. I get quite annoyed by our GP because she doesn't know very much about children with diabetes. I don't ask them anything, but they tell me stuff which is wrong. I actually complained once. I do get my prescriptions from there. He has a supply at school, some here and some at my sister's in case of emergencies.

He's never done a sleepover. People are afraid. There were a handful of people who said they'd have him for a playdate, but we got remarkably few invitations. People didn't know what to do. One friend wrote me a note and offered to do anything, which was very touching. I'll never forget that. It was so generous. I was overwhelmed. I was very aware that others weren't offering.

Mikey pushes boundaries. That's his personality. He does competitive gymnastics and is a showman. When he first meets people, having diabetes makes him a bit cool. Everyone is terribly impressed about his needles and it works well for him. The children go to different schools. We wanted both children to go to the local primary school, but his older brother didn't get in and Mikey did because he had special medical needs.

We also wanted something very nurturing for his older brother, Peter, because there has been so much damage, and he is quite a slow kid. We don't know how profound this is yet, as he is only 10. He finds it difficult to engage with what goes on around him. We've had all sorts of diagnoses, from **autism** to **ADHD** to **dyspraxia**. We've had five different **educational psychology** assessments with five different diagnoses, including 'he's a normal boy', but he is nearly 2 years behind at school. He doesn't verbalise, he didn't talk at all until he was 5, but reads a book a night. I didn't help. I would scream at him daily, I have to accept responsibility for that. He has a lot of support at school, but he has very few friends.

You mustn't give up the fight. You've got to struggle for what you want and you mustn't give up. I know that we have it good compared to others.

Journey collected by Chloe Macaulay, Paediatrician

GLOSSARY

ADHD: Attention deficit hyperactivity disorder.

autism and autistic spectrum disorders: Complex disorders of brain development which affect communication, social interaction and behaviour to varying degrees.

diabetes: A lifelong condition in which blood sugar levels are too high. Childhood-onset diabetes is usually insulin-dependent, meaning that children need lifelong injections of insulin. This means multiple daily injections with regular testing of blood sugar levels. This is done by parents or carers, and by the children themselves when they are old enough. If you have diabetes, you are **'diabetic'**.

dyspraxia: A disorder of physical coordination in which a person can appear clumsy. They can often by helped by the involvement of an occupational therapist and physiotherapist, who can suggest exercises and aids to help.

educational psychology: A branch of psychology that looks at children in an educational environment and at how they learn.

hypo and hyper: Short for *hypoglycaemia* and *hyperglycaemia*, where the blood sugar level is either too low or too high, respectively. Too much insulin can cause hypoglycaemia and too little insulin can cause hyperglycaemia. Both can make one unwell and require action (taking either more sugar or more insulin).

insulin: This is a hormone, produced by the pancreas, that helps to control sugar levels in the body. When sugar levels are high, for example after a meal, insulin is released into the blood stream and brings the sugar level back down. In Type 1 diabetes, the pancreas cannot produce insulin at all and therefore blood sugar levels run very high.

THEMES FOR DISCUSSION

Information and communication
  • Importance of language

Roles and relationships
- Fighting for services
- Expert parents

Diagnosis and clinical care
- Importance of having confidence in staff

Wider impact of illness
- Impact on family life and siblings
- Impact of 'normal' activities like sleepovers

Organisation of care and services
- Education provision

MOLLY

Molly was born at 29 weeks, whilst we were on holiday. The week before, I knew something wasn't right. I could feel she was very low, but my midwife had told me it was safe to go away. At first, I didn't realise I was in labour, but once the pain got really bad, we rushed to hospital and I ended up having an emergency caesarean.

Molly weighed 3 lb 1 oz. Everyone kept telling us she was 'brilliant' and they were convinced we must have got our dates wrong. She was breathing for herself, her skin was in good condition and she was maintaining her own body temperature. We stayed there for 4 days, but the doctors wanted us to return to our local hospital. I was scared. Molly was fine there and I didn't want to move her.

At my local hospital, the nurses wanted me to express some milk for Molly. It was really hard. I was stressed and my body just wasn't producing a lot. The nurses said they'd have to give me tablets to increase my milk production. I felt like I was failing Molly all over again.

Monday was when things went really badly wrong. Andy had to work and I couldn't drive because of the caesarean, so we waited until the afternoon to visit Molly. We knew straight away something had happened. Molly was in a different room by herself and we had to wait outside in the corridor. We could see a nurse sitting really close to her, rubbing her hand. It looked as though Molly had hiccoughs and she was jerking weirdly. Suddenly, we heard them shout for help. Everyone was panicking and I remember Andy saying, 'That's Molly'. No one explained anything to us. We didn't know what was going on and no one asked if we were OK.

We were whisked away into a separate room. A nurse told us they were putting a **long line** in, to give Molly some nutrition, but she was 'misbehaving'. We were left alone in that room, with a box of tissues, for ages. When we did finally see Molly, she looked dreadful and was choking and gasping for air. They decided to 'give her to mum', but I didn't want to hold her for long – she couldn't breathe! Molly was taken away and we thought that was the last time we'd see her.

We went home, but later had to rush back to the hospital as Molly was fitting. She had a tube in her mouth and was all limp and grey. We were in complete shock and didn't know what to do. The doctors couldn't stabilise her. They phoned a specialist hospital for help and a team came to transfer her that night.

The next morning, we went to the specialist hospital where a meeting was being held to discuss Molly. The first thing the consultant said was Molly was breathing for herself, but she had severe brain damage. I remember sitting in that room thinking that our lives have just changed forever.

We learnt that Molly's blood sugar had been off the end of the scale, almost too high to read. The consultant told us that the only time he'd seen something like this was when a child had been given a glucose overdose. They were testing the bags given to Molly, but he said he was sure this wasn't the case here. Already, it felt as though he was trying to protect the other doctors. Little did we know then how right we were. On the ward, Molly did look much better and we were encouraged to touch and hold her. It was such a relief.

Five days later, we were back at our local hospital. They sent us back to the place where everything had gone wrong. Now Molly was known as a 'special' baby because of her brain damage. As soon as we walked into the ward, we noticed a difference. Nurses ignored us and my community midwife would come and see the other babies, but she walked past Molly and me. It was like everyone knew something had happened. Molly's notes weren't kept at the end of her bed like all the other babies. They were kept in the doctor's office.

Molly was born in April and she came home in June, still before her due date. While she had been on the ward, she'd had regular brain scans and we'd seen for ourselves the bleed in her brain getting bigger and bigger. We didn't feel ready to go home.

Over the next few weeks, Molly seemed fairly alert, but she would only look at lights and wouldn't focus on faces. She had a few moments, after the first couple of months, where her head would just drop. It gradually got worse and every time she woke up she made a weird noise and pulled her legs up. One doctor told me she was just coughing. I knew something wasn't right, so I asked to see another doctor who said, 'Well, this is probably the start of it. I think she's having **seizures**'.

After an **EEG**, we were told Molly had a type of epilepsy called **infantile spasms**. I knew it wasn't good news. Before the spasms started, Molly had babbled a lot, but now she was silent. It was horrific, watching her have these attacks. I felt helpless. Molly was prescribed **steroids**, and though they eased the seizures, they didn't stop them. It was getting to the point where I didn't want Molly to wake up because I knew I would just have to sit there, watch her have the seizure and then write it down in the seizure diary. We needed something else.

Just before Molly's first Christmas, we were referred to a specialist children's hospital, where Molly was put on **Epilim**. Her dose was increased gradually until she was nearly 2 years old and on a maximal dose. Though the spasms stopped, Molly was still having **partial seizures**. She slept a lot and looked like a zombie most of the time. By now, we were worried she wasn't developing and wanted the dose reduced. After 4 days of tests, the doctors agreed that Epilim was no longer necessary. When Molly was born, we had been scared to ask the doctors any questions, but now, 2 years later, we had learnt that we had to speak up. We were the only ones who were going to fight for her. Within 2 weeks of being off the Epilim, Molly started to walk.

Molly was supposed to have lots of different people involved in her care as she grew up, because of her special needs, but accessing them was a nightmare. We spent months battling for Molly to have **physiotherapy, speech and language therapy and occupational therapy**. At the age of 3, she was diagnosed with **autism**, but things didn't improve. I felt like I had no say in what went on. People would say 'try this, try that', when really we were just trying to keep our heads above water.

Present Day

Now Molly is nearly 14, her sister Kaitlyn is 17 and their younger brother, Dominic, is 6. We spent the first 10 years of Molly's life fighting a medical negligence case against our local hospital. Molly had been given a massive glucose overdose and the hospital had tried to cover it up by hiding notes and even destroying them.

Life is difficult. Looking after Molly is full on, 24 hours, every single day. She's been ours for nearly 14 years, and yet we're still learning how best to cope. We're trying to have more of a normal life, including Molly in outings, but people don't know how to act around her. All my friends who were pregnant at the same time as me had normal, healthy babies and disappeared when they learnt Molly had 'special needs'. Even Andy's mother has admitted she's scared of her. If we take Molly to hospital, nurses don't want to look after her. She would never hurt a fly, but she can be difficult to manage and they ask us to do everything. We always end up saying, 'Molly's not deaf, she's got special needs'.

We worry a lot about Kaitlyn. It's had a massive effect on her, all through her life. So often, we'd have to drop everything to deal with a Molly crisis and she has consumed our lives. We know Kaitlyn resented Molly. She felt that we loved Molly more than her, as she'd take up so much of our time – especially during the court case. She's come through that difficult patch now, though, and she and Dominic are brilliant. They are very protective of Molly.

Looking back, I was very depressed by it all. I couldn't get my head around it and I would not go back there for all the tea in China. We were on our own, with no help, left to our own devices.

Luckily, because of the court case, we know Molly has the funds to be looked after for the rest of her life. That had been causing us a lot of concern, but now we know she'll be OK. Though we've met some brilliant doctors and nurses along the way, especially when Dominic was born prematurely, we will always be wary. Now we always check things out for ourselves. What happened to Molly was their fault. We know everyone makes mistakes, so if you do, be honest. Never cover it up.

Doctors told us Molly would have no quality of life, that she would be wheelchair bound and wouldn't be able to learn. But she's proving them wrong. She is happy and learning to communicate. Molly loves going for long walks with us, listening to music, playing the piano and spending time on her iPad. She's always laughing and joking.

We wish the mistake hadn't happened – but she is our Molly, all the same.

Journey collected by Felicity Ockelford, medical student

GLOSSARY

autism: A complex disorder of brain development which affects communication, social interaction and behaviour to varying degrees.

EEG: Electroencephalogram – a test used to investigate seizures in which small probes are placed over the head and an electrical tracing of brain activity is taken.

Epilim: The trade name for sodium valproate, a medicine commonly used for the treatment of seizures/epilepsy.

infantile spasms: A type of seizure with characteristic spasmodic movements, seen most commonly in the first year of life. It often has a very poor prognosis.

long line: A form of intravascular access (a long, thin plastic tube inserted into a vein) that is more stable and long-lasting than the normal cannulas used in hospital. It is used when patients need longer-term intravascular access; for example, to provide nutrition through the veins when babies are unable to absorb enough through their guts.

partial seizures: Also known as 'focal seizures', this type of seizure only affects one part of the brain (rather than both hemispheres in a generalised seizure). It can present in a number of different ways depending on which part of the brain is affected; for example, it may cause changes in sensation, lip-smacking, twitching in one part of the body or hallucinations.

physiotherapy, speech and language therapy and occupational therapy: Therapists from these disciplines are all members of the medical multidisciplinary team who work to treat and support patients in a holistic way. Physiotherapists concentrate on physical needs such as helping to clear patients' chests when they have infections or with mobility. Speech and language therapists specialise in assessing speech, language, communication and swallowing. Occupational therapists help and support people to be able to complete day-to-day tasks.

seizure: Also known as a *fit*; a seizure is caused by abnormal electrical activity in the brain and can manifest in a number of different ways, including abnormal movements, usually jerking or sometimes stiffness or stillness.

steroids: A medication that is used for inflammatory conditions. It comes in a number of forms including tablets or creams and may be taken internally or used externally. They also have a role in the management of infantile spasms.

THEMES FOR DISCUSSION

Information and communication
- Listening to/dismissing parental concerns
- Impact of use of words (e.g. 'misbehaving', 'severe brain damage')
- Emergency care/resuscitation – communication with parents – how should it be done?
- Management of birth expectations

Roles and relationships
- Trust

Diagnosis and clinical care
  • Medical errors and how to handle them

Wider impact of illness
  • Effect of chronic illnesses or conditions on siblings
  • Parental mental health and wellbeing
  • Quality of life – what does it mean?

Organisation of care and services
  • Home support for families with children with difficulties such as Molly

RAZA

If I were to start from the beginning, it would mean going back 7 years.

After a year of trying for a baby, I started a treatment called **clomid**, and after two or three courses, I actually became pregnant. We were so excited, crying with happiness. But the next thing that happens is I'm in pain in A&E, and they're telling me there's no baby. It turns out I had an **ectopic pregnancy**.

I tried several different treatments, but nothing worked and we decided to go to Mecca. Within a few months, without any treatment, I became pregnant. I went for a scan at my local hospital and they said, 'We are sorry to tell you, but the baby has no heartbeat'.

With all that happened, I didn't think it would be possible to get pregnant, but 2 months later I was with Raza. I didn't enjoy the pregnancy at all – from the moment I found out to this moment I'm sitting here today, not truly, because as soon as I become happy, something goes wrong. For the first 12 weeks, I didn't tell anyone, not even my own mum. I didn't even want to find out the gender because I felt I would have images of a boy or girl with features of my husband or myself.

Everything seemed to be going OK and then, all of a sudden, I was bleeding heavily. I heard something drop – I assumed I had lost another baby. For 5 weeks I was bleeding. The doctors said there was a threat of miscarriage and I needed to rest. My life came to a complete halt. Luckily, the school I work at was flexible and I stayed at home for the last 6 weeks before school closed for the summer holidays.

At the 20-week scan, things went wrong *again*. The man said he couldn't get a good picture of the heart as the 'baby was lying in a funny position'. In your head, you don't think anything of it, but I had to have follow-up scans and it was clear there were concerns over his heart. We were eventually referred to a specialist centre. That's when they gave it a name – '**tetralogy of Fallot with pulmonary atresia**'. I couldn't even say it, let alone understand what it was.

There were four or five things wrong with him, but after the second I just switched off. Emotionally I couldn't cope. I just couldn't feel anything. I went back to work and one of my colleagues, as usual, said hello and asked how I was. For some reason my heart just burst. I became hysterical. That was the day after they sent the report, so I must have read the letter properly with all the details in black and white and it just got to me. I cried and cried and cried…

Raza was born early at 34 weeks and 5 days. He was screaming when he came out and so at least I knew he was OK. He was born, they lifted him up and he was gone. Within half an hour, the doctor came and asked, 'Has anyone updated you? We have had to **intubate** him as he stopped breathing'.

Within a few days, his condition deteriorated and we were sent to the specialist centre for an urgent operation. They operated and his chest was left open for 4 days because the heart was too swollen to put back in. His heart was literally beating out of his chest, his lips had tripled in size – he didn't feel like my son. When they take consent, they tell you all these stupid dangers and benefits. I remember one of the doctors said there was a possibility that the chest couldn't be closed. Thing is, when they say 'possibility' to you, you don't think it will happen…

Once his chest was closed, his condition improved. We were hoping to move from the intensive care unit to the ward, but that very day he had blood in his stools. He had **necrotising enterocolitis**. I just pretended I couldn't hear it. *Seriously, everything he has faced already, does he need this as well*? I just lost it again. I lost it quite often it seems – I used to cry at everything. Perhaps I was depressed. I saw the paediatric psychotherapist. I poured my heart out to her, but it was Christmas and she had 2 weeks off and so when I was ready to talk to someone, I had no one there.

Here they provide accommodation, but they don't at the local hospital, and it was the most exhausting time of my life. I would go home at 8 p.m., come back at 1 a.m., stay with him until 3 a.m. – it was just too much. Now my husband comes in early and I come in later. I honestly don't know what I would do without him. At one point, it was all too much and I almost left him, but somehow he drew me back in and I can't be more grateful for that. Our marriage has become even stronger. When he is around, I feel like a different person, like my burden is halved.

When you are put into this situation, you have no choice but to be determined for your child. *If he is fighting, why shouldn't you*?

We know that eventually he will have to have another operation, but I'm hoping it's a long while away. I just need him to be a little boy and have a little bit of life before he faces another operation.

Journey collected by Hansini Sivaguru, medical student

GLOSSARY

clomid: Clomiphene citrate, a medication used for fertility treatment for women with polycystic ovaries. It encourages ovulation and carries an increased risk of miscarriage and ectopic pregnancy.

ectopic pregnancy: A pregnancy that develops inside one of the fallopian tubes rather than in the uterus. This can be extremely dangerous for the mother. The pregnancy cannot progress to term and must be removed by surgery.

intubate: Putting a breathing tube (endotracheal tube) down into the lungs to support breathing.

necrotising enterocolitis: A potentially fatal gut condition occurring in new-borns, mostly in premature babies, which requires intensive care management and sometimes surgery. The bowel becomes very inflamed and can become 'necrotic' (dead) and perforate (burst).

tetralogy of Fallot with pulmonary atresia: A congenital cardiac condition (one that a baby is born with) requiring complex surgery, often in the newborn period. The anatomical problems include an abnormal pulmonary artery (the main blood vessel taking blood to the lungs from the heart). The 'pulmonary atresia' mentioned here means that the pulmonary artery was completely closed in Raza's case. Other abnormalities are a ventricular septal defect (hole in the heart), overriding aorta (the main blood vessel carring blood to the body originates in an abnormal place) and right ventricular hypertrophy (thickening of the wall of the right ventricle).

THEMES FOR DISCUSSION

Information and communication
- Information giving
- Breaking bad news

Roles and relationships
- Bonding in the newborn period

Diagnosis and clinical care
- Fertility treatments and its impact
- Care of premature babies

Wider impact of illness
- Being in hospital all the time

Organisation of care and services
- Psychological support available for families

RUBY

Ruby was conceived through **IVF**. It worked the first time and everything seemed fine until about 14 weeks. There was an awful lot of bleeding – I thought I'd miscarried twice. We went to see a private doctor – a professor. He did the **nuchal fold test** and tested my hormone levels, which our council didn't offer at the time. Our risk of having a child with **Down syndrome** came back quite high. He said, 'I'll book you in for a **chorionic villi**'… no question, no discussion, just 'This is what you're gonna do'. We thought, 'This is rubbish, we don't want to do this'. We decided not to. When we told him, he just said, 'What if your baby's got Down's'? We told him we'd get on with it, then he started banging on about how the husbands always go. I said, 'We came to you about bleeding'. He said, 'So what about the bleeding, you bleed like a stuck pig' – unbelievable arrogance. We said, 'Forget it', and we look back at that incident as being very empowering. It's very difficult to resist the pressure of a professor telling you that you need to do something; it's very hard to go against it.

Ruby was born at 28 weeks. She had a straightforward time in **SCBU** – she was only **intubated** for 24 hours. But the routine brain scan showed **flares**. It was quite a scary place because they had some very, very sick babies. You didn't want anyone around your baby's incubator. One day we walked in and there were lots of people around Ruby's incubator… we knew it wasn't good news. The doctor said they'd repeated the **brain ultrasound**, but wouldn't say more. The **neonatologist** gave us a very, very bleak picture. The second scan showed **PVL**. Her prognosis was really poor: she wouldn't see, wouldn't hear, wouldn't speak, wouldn't do anything.

Ruby was diagnosed with **spastic quadriplegic cerebral palsy** by 1 year. We used to go into consultations, but nobody would come out and say it. We used to come out thinking: 'What?!' A **physiotherapist** told us what the diagnosis was in the end. I think they were trying to tell us but they couldn't, it was sort of hinted at rather than spelled out – maybe we were in a state of denial so we weren't listening. The way it was communicated was not the most ideal. People don't like giving bad news.

Somebody once said to me, 'The grieving process never finishes', and I think that's true. It goes on all the time in little steps. It took a while to come to terms with the diagnosis. Initially, it had a major impact on our marriage – we adjusted at different rates and were upset in different ways.

We've got past that. The most important relationship is ours – if we're not alright, Ruby's definitely not – we're aware of that. The best thing of all that the NHS should spend its money on is keeping families together. That's more important than anything. You can have all the different kinds of therapy you want but the breakup of a family is devastating for any child.

We just want Ruby to fulfil her potential, so she can have a nice life. We definitely have to be assertive. It's exhausting, things just move up and down the priority list. You know something's not right, but there are so many other things, you lose sight of it. We're pretty good at getting the equipment we need, but we've had to go through charities and buy stuff privately, and everything costs a fortune. Everything's a battle – we've had to fight for a lot. I had to write to my MP to get things a couple of times. It's funding – I don't want to hear about it – she's entitled to it, why isn't she having it?

We built our house; it's specially adapted for Ruby, all level access. Ruby is going to live here. The upstairs bit is our bedroom, but ultimately a carer can live there. We've written a will and set up a trust for her. I worry about the future constantly, you just end up going nuts actually.

Ruby's condition is global, so there are lots of people involved. Dealing with many, many specialists is hard. We act as the fulcrum of it all. They say they're in contact – copying and forwarding reports – that's their integration. Often, they read the reports when you're sat in the appointment. We end up having the same conversations over and over. Ruby has started her second lever arch file at hospital. I sometimes think to myself, 'This is a lifetime, where are they going to put all her notes'? But people only ever seem to refer to the top few.

Dealing with the paperwork is a huge job; for example, the application form for **DLA**, it's massive! It's emotional and insulting, why are we having to do it so regularly?

Ruby's patient journey is ongoing, with multiple touch points, all the time. You could argue it's not a journey for us, because there's no end destination. It's a way of life.

Journey collected by Poppy Redman, medical student

GLOSSARY

brain ultrasound (also known as a cranial ultrasound scan): This is an investigation that is commonly performed on the neonatal unit, where an ultrasound scan is performed of the baby's brain by placing some jelly and a probe on the baby's fontanelle (soft spot). It allows doctors to see the basic anatomy of the brain and determine whether there are any problems like bleeding or enlargement of the ventricles ('water spaces') of the brain.

chorionic villi: Refers to chorionic villus sampling, a procedure performed antenatally (before birth) in which a sample of placental tissue is taken in order to look for chromosomal abnormalities in the foetus.

DLA: Disability Living Allowance. A benefit available to families/patients with certain long term conditions or disabilites.

Down syndrome: A congenital condition caused by having three copies of chromosome 21 instead of two ('trisomy 21'). It is associated with characteristic facial features, learning difficulty and often other problems, such as heart and gut defects and thyroid disease.

flares: Bright areas seen on a cranial ultrasound scan. The presence of flares does not usually mean anything on its own, but flares are monitored with further scans to watch how they develop.

intubated: Where a breathing tube (endotracheal tube) has been put down into the baby's lungs to support his or her breathing.

IVF: In vitro fertilisation; a process by which the female's egg is fertilised by the male's sperm outside the body and then implanted into the female.

neonatologist: A doctor who specialises in newborn babies.

nuchal fold test: During an antenatal scan (an ultrasound scan performed on a pregnant woman), measurements are taken of the thickness of the 'nuchal fold' – the fat at the back of the unborn baby's neck. This measurement can give an indication of the risk of the baby having certain conditions such as Down syndrome and is used as a screening test.

physiotherapist: A professional who specialises in supporting patients with their physical needs; for example, building up strength and improving mobility.

PVL: 'Periventricular leukomalacia' – damage to areas of white matter in the brain, which can cause characteristic appearances on a head scan. It occurs most commonly in very preterm infants due to decreased blood and oxygen supply to parts of the brain and is usually associated with a poor developmental outcome. Babies with PVL may develop cerebral palsy.

SCBU: Special care baby unit – a unit in which unwell and/or premature babies are looked after.

spastic quadriplegic cerebral palsy: Cerebral palsy is a disorder of movement and posture caused by an insult to the developing brain which can happen before, during or after birth. It can affect children in a number of different ways and varies greatly in severity from very mild to very severe. Ruby has 'spastic quadriplegic cerebral palsy', which means that she has increased tone in all four of her limbs and is likely to have poor head control. This type of cerebral palsy is also associated with seizures. Children with this form of cerebral palsy usually need help with all daily activities, including feeding, washing and moving.

THEMES FOR DISCUSSION

Information and communication
- Breaking bad news

Roles and relationships
- Paternalism

Diagnosis and clinical care
- Impact of diagnosis

Wider impact of illness
- Living with uncertainty and uncertain futures
- Supporting families
- 'Grieving' for a child with a chronic illness

Organisation of care and services
- DLA and funding for children with disabilities

SELENA

I was born in a small village in Cameroon 17 years ago and didn't realise that I had **HIV** until my mum told me, when I wasn't yet 13. My mum didn't know that either of us were infected until she moved to the UK when I was around 2 years old. My parents moved to find better jobs to help support family members back in Cameroon and to find a better life for me.

Because of the healthcare system where I was born, my mother wasn't screened for the virus and there was poor access to formula milk, so I was breastfed. She didn't even know that that could increase the chances of transmission. Along with a natural delivery, the chances of me getting HIV were pretty high.

I was a bit of a sickly child. Apparently, a couple of months after I was born, I'd had swollen glands and recurrent ear infections, but the doctors in Cameroon didn't think it was anything serious. They sent me home without doing any further investigations into the cause of my illnesses. Shortly after we arrived in the UK, my mum took me to the doctor because I had a bad fever and cough and wouldn't stop crying. I also had a funny-looking rash on my back. The doctor noted that I wasn't growing as would be expected of a child my age and he got suspicious. He asked my mum about HIV and she agreed for us both to be tested. As it turns out, we were both positive.

I don't know my dad. He refused to be tested and my mum left him as soon as she found out that she was HIV positive because she knew that he'd given it to her and she'd given it to me as a result. To this day, he doesn't know about my diagnosis. In actual fact, nobody does – just me and Mum. I have a little brother who's negative and even he doesn't know. Mum says that she doesn't want people to know because they'll treat me differently.

Sometimes it's really hard to keep it to myself and I feel like I'm going to explode if I don't tell anyone. But when I get really close to someone and feel like telling them, I get absolutely terrified that they'll be scared of touching me and treat me like a leper. The doctors encourage me to find a friend that I trust and let them know, but I just can't do it. I'm also scared of what my mum will do if she finds out I've let anyone know. She's tried so hard to keep it a secret for such a long time. She even brought a magazine to the doctor's that had an article in it called *My Mum Gave Me HIV!* to prove how sensational these revelations can be. They aren't treated by the public as unfortunate events that happen to real people, they are considered travesties with someone who needs to be blamed.

I was referred to the children's hospital pretty much immediately and I was in a bad way. My **viral load** was high and my **CD4⁺ cell count** dropping steadily. The doctors told me years later that if they hadn't found out when they did, I would have had **AIDS** within a year and died. This was when I was finally told about my disease. Apparently, the doctors had been trying to get my mum to tell me about the HIV since I was around 8. It took ten visits before she finally told me why we'd been going to the doctor my whole life.

I feel like I always knew something serious was wrong with me, despite being told by Mum that I was just a little sick. Even if I had known what HIV was, the clinic at the hospital is called the ABC clinic to protect people's confidentiality and the school gets special letters that don't tell them why I have to miss lessons now and then, so I would never have known. Now that my brother's 10, the doctors have been trying to get Mum to disclose our HIV status to him and teach him about the risks of transmission, but she's adamant that she doesn't want him to know, for a few years at the very least. I know that she's just trying to protect us all, but I feel like he might suspect something eventually, just like I did when I was younger. I don't want it to cause any problems, but there's always that little part of me that's afraid he'll treat me differently when he finds out.

Nowadays, my viral load is undetectable and I have a healthy CD4⁺ cell count thanks to the doctors and nurses, and I try to lead as normal a life as possible. I only have to take two pills a day, **AZT and nevirapine**, which isn't too difficult, and the doctors say that my compliance is why my disease is so well controlled. It wasn't always like this though. When I was 15, I got quite depressed and stopped taking my medication every day. I had to go to hospital because I got a cough that turned out to be **bacterial pneumonia**. The doctors were disappointed with me, but it had just got to a point where I felt sick of having my life controlled by a disease that wasn't even my fault. I snapped and told Mum this when she asked me why I did it and she cried for a long time. I felt awful and started to take my medication again and eventually got back to where I was before. I still feel like I will always be labelled as a 'sufferer' of HIV, and that makes me feel like I have less potential in life than someone who is 'normal', but I know that it's important that I comply with treatment or I'll have no life at all.

Now that I'm 17, the team at the children's hospital have started to mention transitioning to adult services. The transition nurse is really nice and friendly and took me to the young persons' clinic to show me around and has been teaching me about safe sex and how to book appointments on my own. The young persons' clinic was different but it seemed OK. There were people my own age there, and knowing that I'm not alone in this makes me feel a bit better about moving than if I just went straight into an adult clinic. I just feel really sad that as soon as I'm 18, it's out the door. Goodbye. The nurse that first saw me when I came here still sees me now and we always talk for a while when she has time. She asks me about school and my life and sees me as a person, not as a disease. She's like family to me now; they all are. It feels like my parents are kicking me out of the house because they've got a new kid they have to look after now. It's not the doctors' or nurses' fault, it's the system's, but I'm not ready to go yet. When I look at my mum when they mention transition, she looks even more upset than I feel. I think that even though she has her own doctors, the team here are sort of a support network for her, a second parent to me. After all, they've practically helped raise me.

When I used to think about the future, all I saw was a miserable, unfulfilled life, but I don't feel that way anymore. My mind automatically jumped to conclusions of being unable to have a husband that loved me for who I was, being unable to have children and dying early. The doctors spent a long time trying to reassure me and, at first, I didn't believe them. I did my own research and found out that it really is true. HIV-positive women can have children if enough precautions are taken, and if I comply with my medication, I can live to a similar age as a person without the disease. I have blips now and then where I feel sad and wonder why my mother and I had to be affected by this terrible disease, but ultimately, I know that if we stay strong, we can help each other to be happy. When I think about it, I have a lot to be grateful for: a good education, a loving mother and a fantastic team of doctors and nurses who I owe so much to.

Journey collected by James Williams, medical student

GLOSSARY

AIDS: Acquired immunodeficiency syndrome – the latter stages of symptoms of HIV infection where the immune system is no longer working properly and the patient is susceptible to potentially life-threatening infections that are caused by bacteria and viruses that would not normally make those with healthy immune systems unwell. People with AIDS are also more likely to develop certain types of cancer and can have symptoms such as fever, swollen glands and diarrhoea. Not everyone with HIV will develop AIDS.

AZT and nevirapine: These are two types of antiretroviral drugs (medications used to treat HIV and AIDS). These treatments are most commonly given in combination rather than one drug alone, as this tends to be more effective at treating HIV.

bacterial pneumonia: A bacterial infection of the lungs that requires treatment with antibiotics.

CD4$^+$ cell count: A measure of how much the HIV is affecting the immune system and is used alongside the viral load to decide on the treatment plan. In well-controlled patients, the count will be high.

HIV: Human immunodeficiency virus – virus that attacks the immune system, leaving it less able to fight infections and other diseases such as certain types of cancer. It is most commonly acquired through unprotected sex, but can also be acquired through blood contact such as sharing needles for injection or blood transfusions and transfer from mother to baby during pregnancy, child birth or breastfeeding. There is no cure, but with good compliance to treatment, many people with HIV can live a long and healthy life.

viral load: A measure of the amount of HIV in the blood. This is monitored to help with decisions regarding when patients need to start on treatment and how effective the treatment is. When patients are well controlled, the viral load is low, and this means that they are much less likely to pass on infection to anyone else.

FURTHER READING

HIV and AIDS, nhs.uk. http://www.nhs.uk/Conditions/HIV/Pages/Introduction.aspx

THEMES FOR DISCUSSION

Information and communication
- When to tell: keeping diagnoses from children

Roles and relationships
- Being seen as a person, not a disease
- Confidentiality and respecting families' wishes

Diagnosis and clinical care
- Compliance with treatment
- Transition to adult care

Wider impact of illness
- Labels and stigma
- Psychological impact of life-long conditions
- The challenges of being a 'normal' teenager

Organisation of care and services
- Healthcare in developing countries

TOMMY

Tommy was born normally at term, but once he came home, he had great difficulties in breastfeeding and I began to suffer from mastitis. The GP then told me to stop breastfeeding immediately and Tommy had to go onto formula. He was still very unhappy about feeding, but the GP said that this was probably because he was a hungry baby and needed a higher fat content. My instincts told me this couldn't be right, but he was the GP, and I was a first-time mum, so I went along with his advice and changed formula again.

Whilst trying these different feeds, Tommy developed **cradle cap** at the top of his forehead and this kept spreading. The midwife suggested we try olive oil and water, which we did. But it then started spreading from the neck to the chest. So, again, we went back to the GP. He said Tommy may have infantile eczema, so we were given creams and swapped to soya milk. Then he developed a **staphylococcal infection**. He looked so sore, as if he had been scalded, so we decided to take him to hospital. He was only 4 weeks old at this point and we were worried.

Since we went to a training hospital, we saw different consultants daily, and the lack of continuity of care led to conflicting diagnoses being given by the different consultants. He was then given another milk that was supposed to be easier to digest, which made him very sick, and he suffered from diarrhoea because of the side effects of his antibiotics. Five days into the antibiotic course, they were talking about sending him home. The problem was, everything he was taking came straight back out again. He vomited on the car journey home, so we went straight back to hospital. They kept telling us it was due to **reflux** and infantile diarrhoea, but Tommy wasn't sleeping like my friends' babies; when he tried to empty his bowels he used to scream in pain, and the sickness and diarrhoea were relentless.

This was when I decided to do my own research. I read on a website that there could be a link between the bowel and skin problems, which suggested using a different kind of milk. Armed with this information and a family member for support, I went back to the hospital and showed the doctor. He said that they would do more tests, but we were fed up of having more tests done. Right on cue, Tommy vomited on the floor. I think this made the doctor realise our suspicions that there was something seriously wrong with Tommy. I insisted he needed to see a paediatric gastroenterologist; he was 6 months old and failing to thrive, and his dad and I had been sleeping in shifts for the last 6 months. The consultant acceded and referred him to the children's hospital.

We noted all the information about Tommy down, including all the medications and formula milks we had tried; we had fought to get ourselves to the children's hospital, so didn't want to be seen to be wasting the doctor's time there. The doctor realised that Tommy's case was very serious, so gave him a higher dose of **ranitidine**, but this didn't stop the vomiting or diarrhoea. Eventually, Tommy had an **endoscopy**. He also had a **biopsy**, which gave him a diagnosis – a condition that, at the time, was only recognised at this hospital, **eosinophilic gastroenterocolitis**. Some doctors don't believe this condition exists, but if you have met Tommy, you will know that it does.

Tommy is now in Year 6, although he hasn't been to school since September. If he gets a virus, it triggers everything off and his body can flare up. This means that he has to be admitted to hospital to go on gut rest and is only fed **intravenously**. But we had to wait 3 months to get a bed here, and in that time, he lost a quarter of his body weight. The nutrition he gets is from **elemental feeds**, and any food he has is only to keep his digestive tract motile; he has **malabsorption**, so obtains no nutritional benefit from it.

We have had to fight for a **statement of special educational needs**. Luckily, I have the support of my husband, otherwise I don't know what I would have done. I still don't think the school understands how this condition affects Tommy; this is the problem with a condition that you can't touch and can't see. Since he has significant abdominal pain, he has never been able to sleep well at night, so struggles to concentrate at school. The bedwetting doesn't bother him, it is just the abdominal pain – his pain level never goes below 5/10.

We also have a daughter, Amy. She also suffers from this condition, but has different symptoms to Tommy. We say that we don't know what to do, but we know what not to do, based on our experiences with Tommy. We don't introduce two foods at once, as no food is asymptomatic.

Being a rare condition, we didn't realise it was genetic, and it is heart-breaking for me to see Amy suffering as well. I don't know whether we would have had Amy had we known, but I cannot imagine my life without her, and hopefully Tommy always has someone who understands what he is going through. Sometimes, it can be hard to mother her; in the 5 weeks in which Tommy has been in hospital, I have only seen Amy for a day. I have also had to give up my work; looking after my children is now my full-time job.

We have learnt to throw out any rules that one has about the human body, as Tommy and Amy's bodies work in exactly the opposite way. We also tell one another that we are normal until we leave the house; our normal is not other peoples' normal, but we are perfectly happy with that.

Journey collected by Shivan Kotecha, medical student

GLOSSARY

biopsy: Where a sample of tissue is taken for analysis in order to aid diagnosis.

cradle cap: A common and generally harmless skin problem in babies in which the scalp and sometimes the face become scaly.

elemental feeds: A liquid feed taken by mouth or straight into the stomach via a nasogastric tube or gastrostomy, which contains all of the essential dietary requirements in a broken down form to allow for easy digestion.

endoscopy: An investigation in which a long scope with a camera on the end is inserted into the bowel, either via the mouth or up the bottom (in this case the mouth), in order to visualise the inside of the bowel. Samples of the bowel ('biopsies') can be taken at the same time. This can be used in order to diagnose or monitor disease within the bowel.

eosinophilic gastroenterocolitis: A condition causing gut inflammation and gastrointestinal symptoms. The diagnosis is made on the basis of gut symptoms and gut inflammation and eosinophilic infiltration on biopsy (eosinophils are a type of white cell).

intravenously: Through the veins.

malabsorption: When the gut fails to properly absorb nutrients from food across the gut wall, which can lead to failure to thrive and deficiencies.

ranitidine: A medication used to suppress acid production in the stomach.

reflux: Gastro-oesophageal reflux, in which the stomach contents (food and/or acid) come back up the oesophagus (feeding tube) and can cause discomfort and vomiting. This is more common in babies, as the connection between the stomach and oesophagus is floppier and they also spend more time on their backs (making it easier for milk to flow back up).

staphylococcal infection: Staphylococci are bacteria that can cause different types of infection of variable severity, commonly in the skin, requiring antibiotic treatment.

statement of special educational needs: A formal document that outlines a child's needs and the support that should be given to them when they have a condition that affects their ability to learn. This has been replaced by an Education Health Plan.

THEMES FOR DISCUSSION

Information and communication
- Parental sources of information/research

Roles and relationships
- Being a 'first-time mum'

Diagnosis and clinical care
- Continuity of care
- Rare conditions and their wider impact

Wider impact of illness
- Effect on schooling
- Impact on siblings
- Adjusting to a 'new normal'

Organisation of care and services
- Role of specialist versus local hospitals
- Special educational needs provision

WENDY

There was nothing special about the pregnancy. I think we just expected everything to be normal. I seem to remember my wife was prescribed something for heartburn. We were more comfortable with those small things this time. This was our second child, Wendy. Our first child was just 13 months old when Wendy was born.

During the first pregnancy, we needed an emergency caesarean section and my wife **haemorrhaged**. Coming out of that experience, we were sure that there was nothing worse that could be thrown at us. Then, when 29 weeks pregnant with Wendy, my wife began having trouble breathing, so we went straight to hospital. An ultrasound scan revealed that the baby was in breech position. Although we had intended on a natural birth, the doctors started planning another caesarean.

Wendy was born at 39 weeks gestation. After being in recovery with my wife, we were taken to see our new baby. There was a **paediatric nurse** waiting for us there. That was when we knew that something wasn't right. Wendy's midface was folded inwards. I couldn't even see her eyes. I wasn't sure she had eyes. This should be one of the happiest times of your life, but instead we were just so worried. The nurse told us that she might be blind and deaf. They used lots of medical words to explain, but all we heard was blind and deaf.

Over the next 36 hours, we saw a **paediatrician** and an eye specialist. We were told that one eye looked normal, and that she was likely to be blind in the other. I felt like Wendy's face changed a lot during that time. The tip of her nose seemed to come down and her eyes became visible beneath her brow. Still, I badgered the doctor with questions. I remember hearing that they thought it was a kind of syndrome, so I made the doctor tell me exactly. He suggested something called **Treacher–Collins syndrome**. Looking it up on the internet scared us a bit. Since then, we have tried to avoid looking up conditions that the doctors mention straight away.

We left hospital on the third day. Nevertheless, for at least the next week, we returned every day. Although it was primarily an eye problem, the hospital thought there could be other abnormalities internally. I don't like the word 'abnormality' much though: it has such negative connotations. Wendy's eye was also reviewed and we were referred to the children's hospital to have further investigations. Wendy was still less than a month old.

In the meantime, she wasn't putting on any weight, so the health visitor was coming around to check on her. We noticed that she was crying and distressed when trying to defecate, so we visited the GP for advice. During the appointments, Wendy was asleep. The doctor just said that crying was normal. I felt a bit like he had fobbed us off.

Near to Christmas, I noticed Wendy's eye starting to bulge. Our hospital pushed for an emergency appointment at the children's hospital. The surgeon there cancelled his holiday and they operated on Christmas Eve. When I thanked him, he said it was no trouble, and that he would probably never see a case like this again. He said, 'This is why I do my job'.

We returned in the New Year to review Wendy's eye. They planned a whole course of surgeries. Three days later, she was having a **cornea transplant** and the beginnings of eyelid reconstruction. That night, Wendy was very unhappy. When the doctor came to check on us, she passed a stool with blood in it. She was back in surgery again the next morning. The surgery was really long, and the longer it was, the more worried we became. As updates came to us during the procedure, it was explained that Wendy had something called **necrotising enterocolitis**. Afterwards, we were informed that a large part of her bowel was removed and she had been given a **stoma**.

She was placed in intensive care. It's a scary place for someone non-medical. The worst part was that Wendy needed to be sedated there for almost a week. When she recovered, we were sent to the high dependency unit. Soon after, I noticed a bulge in her bandage. I peeled it back to find an open wound. I pulled the emergency cord by her bed and the surgical ward round going on next door descended on our room. We were back in surgery within 15 minutes. The staff explained the operation and took consent on the way to the theatre. We had our own nurse looking after us throughout the surgery. My wife cried and I was sick.

After, she was put on a special machine by the **tissue viability team** to encourage skin growth where the wound was. It was still undergoing research, but to be honest, I would have signed anything at that point. The hospital put Wendy onto **total parenteral nutrition** and she's gradually getting back to normal. I'm glad that we're now in charge of Wendy's eye care too. You tend to feel quite useless while hospital staff look after your child all day.

Fortunately, my work allowed me time off to stay with Wendy, but not everyone is so lucky. Her room has a bed for a parent to stay in overnight.

It's reassuring for us and the nurses to know that there's always someone there with Wendy. The only downside is leaving our firstborn with her grandparents. I think she was just starting to get used to her new sister. She is growing up so fast that whenever I'm home, she likes different foods and plays with different toys.

Wendy is almost 3 months old and has three major surgeries behind her. There are four operations left. Hopefully, we will soon be at home, as a family in one place again.

Journey collected by Alex Harper, medical student

GLOSSARY

cornea transplant: The cornea is the transparent covering over the front of the eye. In a transplant, the damaged cornea is removed and replaced with a new 'graft' made from healthy donor tissue.

haemorrhaged: Meaning bled heavily.

necrotising enterocolitis: A gut condition occurring in newborns, mostly in premature babies, which requires intensive care management and sometimes surgery. The bowel becomes very inflamed and can become 'necrotic' (dead) and perforate (burst). It can be fatal.

paediatric nurse: A nurse specialising in children and young people.

paediatrician: A doctor specialising in the health of children and young people.

stoma: Part of the bowel that is brought out to the surface of the skin, either to let the bowel below heal or because it is not possible to reconnect it. Depending on what type of stoma it is, a bag may be put over it to collect the effluent coming out. They can be temporary or permanent.

tissue viability team: A specialised team that manages vulnerable skin and wounds.

total parenteral nutrition: 'Liquid nutrition' administered through the veins when feeding through the normal enteral route is either not possible or inadequate for meeting the child's needs.

Treacher–Collins syndrome: A rare syndrome affecting the bones and soft tissues of the face. There is a large spectrum of severity.

THEMES FOR DISCUSSION

Information and communication
- Breaking bad news
- The impact of words: deaf, blind, abnormality
- The internet as a source of information

Roles and relationships
- Parental feeling of helplessness/lack of control

Diagnosis and clinical care
- Hospital experience
- Intensive care experience

Wider impact of illness
- Impact on family

Organisation of care and services
- Primary versus secondary versus tertiary services

3

Themes for Discussion

Chloe Macaulay, Polly Powell and Caroline Fertleman

This section summarises some of the themes that arise from the different patient journeys. It is not in anyway exhaustive but can be used as a prompt to aid discussion and reflection.

Themes	Aasif	Abbey	Ashoka	Ava
Information and communication	• Parental intuition	• Advantages and disadvantages of different types of communication (e.g. lost letters, telephone calls, etc.) • Failure to communicate important information – why this might happen	• Checking understanding	• Sources of information
Roles and relationships	• Different family roles • Family members as carers	• Trust • Being a father versus being a mother (e.g. in the NICU)	• Accepting doctors' reassurances • Taking responsibility for yourself • Parents as organ donors for their children	• Importance of establishing who the carer is
Diagnosis and clinical care	• Genetic counselling and testing • The 'relief' of receiving a definite diagnosis	• Missing a diagnosis – why this might happen and how it could be dealt with	• Diagnostic tests available in different places	• Sensory impairment
Wider impact of illness	• How illnesses are perceived in different cultures and religions • Helping children with medical conditions to integrate	• Effect of stillbirth/miscarriage • How different people deal with loss	• Migration for health reasons • Accepting a new normality • Effect on friendships	
Organisation of care and services	• Financial help available to families • Special schools	• How different hospitals work (e.g. allowing parents to be present while staff handover the patients versus asking them to leave)	• Healthcare in developing countries • Transition to adult services	• MDTs • Special schools • Looked-after children

Abbreviations: NICU: neonatal intensive care unit; MDT: multidisciplinary team.

Themes	David	Dillon	Ella	Harry
Information and communication	• Breaking bad news	• Breaking bad news • Communication between teams	• Use of jargon/acronyms (e.g. JDM) • The internet as a source of information	• Dealing with uncertainty ('wait and see')
Roles and relationships	• Support for cancer patients • The parent's role as advocate for the child	• Dealing with different teams • The parent as advocate • Emotional attachment of staff	• Listening to parents	• Family dynamics • Relationships with health professionals
Diagnosis and clinical care	• Cancer treatment • Aggressive versus palliative treatment – when to stop • Do not resuscitate orders	• The journey to a diagnosis	• The hospital experience	• Impact of a diagnosis such as cerebral palsy and what it means to others
Wider impact of illness	• 'Not giving up'	• Wider family impact	• Losing your identity as a person • Impact on parents (e.g. stress; prolonged separation)	• Social implications of having a chronically unwell child (e.g. for holidays)
Organisation of care and services	• Palliative care services	• End-of-life care	• Local versus specialist services	• Educational provision for children with special needs • Transitioning to adult care

Abbreviation: JDM: juvenile dermatomyositis.

Themes	Henry	Jo	Katy	Laura
Information and communication	• Impact of words such as 'meningitis' • Explaining conditions to family members • Media depiction of health services	• Use of words	• Non-verbal communication • Communication between teams	• 'Reading up' on conditions and sources of information
Roles and relationships	• Challenging a doctor's decisions • Supporting role of medical staff	• Parental roles	• 'Expert parents' • Team working • Support for families	• Trust in medical profession
Diagnosis and clinical care	• Behavioural change and psychological diagnoses versus physical diagnoses	• Safeguarding procedures	• Uncertainty	• The 'need' to separate babies from their mothers after caesarean section if babies need to go to neonatal intensive care
Wider impact of illness	• Attitudes and experiences of disability • Effect on siblings • Taking each day as it comes	• Reactions to accidents and life-changing events	• Impact on family life	• Impact of a stillbirth • Impact of death and illness on families, siblings and marital relationships
Organisation of care and services		• Organisation of emergency services and departments • Local versus specialist units • Visiting and sleeping arrangements for families	• Coordination between teams and services	• Autopsies for stillbirths • Tertiary neonatal units (level 3) versus local neonatal units (levels 1–2)

Themes	Lily	Luke	Mikey	Molly
Information and communication	• Understanding risks and benefits of treatment	• Impact of words such as 'oncology', and statistics • How much information to give	• Importance of language	• Listening to/dismissing parental concerns • Impact of use of words (e.g. 'misbehaving' and 'severe brain damage') • Emergency care/resuscitation; communication with parents; how should it be done? • Management of birth expectations
Roles and relationships	• Medicalisation of families and the expert parent	• Autonomy and consent in young people/adolescence • Having a sibling with cancer • The 'expert patient' • Paternalism	• Fighting for services • Expert parents	• Trust
Diagnosis and clinical care	• Rare conditions • Intensive care settings	• Long term effects of cancer treatments	• Importance of having confidence in staff	• Medical errors and how to handle them
Wider impact of illness	• How families adapt • Effect on siblings	• Physical stigmata of certain conditions, for example losing your hair • Being a teenager with a long term condition (LTC)	• Impact on family life and siblings • Impact on 'normal' activities like sleepovers	• Effect of chronic illnesses or conditions on siblings • Parental mental health and wellbeing • Quality of life – what does it mean?
Organisation of care and services	• Schooling for ill children	• Financial support available for families with children with LTCs	• Educational provision	• Home support for families with children with difficulties

Themes	Raza	Ruby	Selena	Tommy
Information and communication	• Information giving • Breaking bad news	• Breaking bad news	• When to tell: keeping diagnoses from children	• Parental sources of information/research
Roles and relationships	• Bonding in the newborn period	• Paternalism	• Being seen as a person, not a disease • Confidentiality and respecting families' wishes	• Being a 'first-time mum'
Diagnosis and clinical care	• Fertility treatments and its impact • Care of premature babies	• Impact of diagnosis	• Compliance with treatment • Transition to adult care	• Continuity of care • Rare conditions and their wider impacts
Wider impact of illness	• Being in hospital all the time	• Living with uncertainty and uncertain futures • Supporting families • 'Grieving' for a child with a chronic illness	• Labels and stigma • Psychological impact of life-long condition • The challenges of being a 'normal' teenager	• Effect on schooling • Impact on siblings • Adjusting to a new 'normal'
Organisation of care and services	• Psychological support available for families	• DLA and funding for children with disabilities	• Healthcare in developing countries	• Role of specialist versus local hospitals • Special educational need provision

Abbreviation: DLA: Disability Living Allowance.

Themes	Wendy
Information and communication	• Breaking bad news • The impact of words ('deaf', 'blind' and 'abnormality') • The internet as a source of information
Roles and relationships	• Parental feeling of helplessness/lack of control
Diagnosis and clinical care	• Hospital experience • Intensive care experience
Wider impact of illness	• Impact on family
Organisation of care and services	• Primary care versus secondary care versus tertiary care

4

Reflections on Learning through Patient Journeys

Bryony Alderman

Journey – a process of travelling from one place to another. Inherent in the word is a sense of ongoing, something long lasting, perhaps convoluted and challenging at times.

In the medical profession, encounters with patients can easily be viewed as discrete events, with a clear beginning and end. One can forget that patients' experiences and thoughts about their healthcare persist and progress. They do not end once the consulting room door swings closed, or when the jostling ward round moves on to the next bed.

For this reason, the concept of the patient journey is an important one, emphasising the continuous nature of healthcare, its pervasiveness and its potential for challenges, complexity and wrong turns.

As a doctor in the very early stages of my career, I know I still have a great deal to learn. I used patient stories – generously provided by the families who had experienced them – as an educational tool before I had even started my formal clinical training, when the image of myself as a doctor was unimaginably distant. These 'journeys' were a novel way of prompting discussion and promoting understanding of the patient perspective in a safe and supportive environment.

From my personal experience as a healthcare professional in training, it is often inevitable to become tied up in critical assessment of oneself when learning to consult with patients. Did I ask the right set of questions to rule out this or that differential? Was my tone of voice appropriate? Did I show empathy, build rapport, listen appropriately and pick up on my patient's cues?

Important as this reflection is for improving practice, such a stream of internal questioning can detract from thinking about patients themselves, and in the limited time available in a busy healthcare setting, it is not often that one is afforded the luxury of a patient or family's full narrative, and this was the first benefit of learning through patient journeys.

Before writing this piece, I looked back through notes and essays I had drafted as a student whilst studying the stories we had been given. Even now, some of the diagnoses and clinical histories are more complex than the usual preserve of a junior doctor. But the utility of the discussion went far beyond learning stark facts about rare conditions. What was striking was that even a limited understanding of history, examination and diagnosis did not in any way prevent me from engaging with the human aspects of medicine that these stories presented. You don't need to know the meaning of every test result or investigation to be able to explore the impact of experiences on patients and their families. To quote William Osler (1849–1919), 'The good physician treats the disease; the great physician treats the patient who has the disease'. The appreciation of *people* is for me what underpins medical practice, and learning to take an interest in thoughts and feelings before learning symptoms and signs was a solid foundation for my future practice.

It is extraordinary to witness the common themes that arose in numerous stories that my classmates and I discussed, such as dealing with uncertainty – for example, poor communication – the confusion of seeing multiple professionals and the conflicting views they could offer. Finding these common threads through the study of patient journeys helped to cement them in my mind, and I try even now to pay them due attention.

Studying the patient journey, using the stories that have been generously shared by those who have had such experiences, can provide healthcare professionals with food for thought, teaching them to look outside of the consultation room and see that their own encounter with a patient may occupy but a tiny space within a rich odyssey. By having the luxury of hearing first-hand patient experiences, maybe we can become more accepting of this role, while at the same time ensuring that we give our best to each patient in order to facilitate their onward journey.

5

Getting in Touch: Reflections on Clinical Attentiveness

Sebastian Kraemer

Though physical contact is a common element in many clinical encounters, this chapter is about the extent to which our minds can match our hands, and get in touch with the patient's experience.

PATIENT JOURNEYS: PRACTICE AND THEORY

Group discussion of clinical narratives is a powerful method of learning. Members have to put themselves in the patient's or parent's shoes and at the same time accept that their peers see it differently. Unlike in a classroom, there are no right answers. All perceptions are equally useful for exploration by the group. When this kind of reflection is encouraged, students discover just how expert they can be at identifying with other people. This is not technical knowledge such as 'psychology' or 'communication skills'; it is a capacity we all began to learn before we could talk.

Your experience of being looked after as a child strongly influences the way you relate with and care for others: your friends, colleagues, partner, children and patients. Identification is a basic and necessary human skill, without which our contact with patients and families would be very limited. Patient journey seminars activate ordinary personal qualities that can then be integrated into clinical work. How did we acquire these? Until the twentieth century, there was little scientific understanding of child development. Then rival theories began to argue over the relative importance of learning on the one hand and of love and hate on the other. This was a great step forward, but it was not until the 1960s that biology and psychology were brought together in attachment theory,[1,2] which began to demonstrate the primary drive for protection in all mammals, which is quite distinct from the need to be fed. We can readily see it in farm animals, such as lambs, who always rush to the ewe when someone approaches.

Seeking help from health services highlights our life-long attachment needs. At birth, humans are the most immature of all mammals and have a much longer period of helplessness. During this time, mind and brain develop according to the experience of care that the child receives. At first, the child is totally unable to look after him or herself, and has no sense of time, only of the presence or absence of a caregiver whom he or she attracts with smiles or by crying. Despite the absence of predators in most modern human settings, a tiny child is fearful of abandonment and very sensitive to how you handle him or her. The people doing the looking after – parents, grandparents, childminders and others – are most helpful once the child gets to know and trust them, and this works best when they know and trust each other too.

The term 'good enough mother'[3] was coined to highlight the fact that a caregiver cannot possibly be in perfect sync with a baby. She may be too close or too far away, speak too loudly or be too hurried or too slow, and has to learn by trial and error how best to be in touch with the child. This is how infants learn about time, and about hope. If the people looking after you in the early years take you seriously as a person in your own right, with a mind – and a sense of humour – of your own, then your brain gets wired up to be curious about and interested in others' experiences, precisely because that has happened to you.[4] A secure attachment sets the body's psychology and physiology in balance, protecting the child from overreacting to the normal stresses of life and preparing him or her for future relationships of all kinds. If caregivers are too often out of touch, then the child's development adapts to that, and he or she grows up either denying any need for help ('I'll just have to manage on my own') or anxiously seeking it but then not being able to receive it.

Both patient and clinician bring their attachment experiences to the consultation. The patient has learned over a lifetime how much hope and trust it is safe to put into anyone who is trying to help. In turn, using your own life-long learning, the best you can achieve is to be a good enough practitioner. It is not patronising to think of clinical care in terms of attachment. Whatever their age, anyone who needs help will show something of their habitual way of seeking it. In every clinical encounter, we have to find the right emotional distance to understand and be understood.

- Being ill or in need of help activates attachment behaviours at any stage of life.
- Patients' expectations of you are conditioned by the kinds of care they received in the past in their own families and when seeking help from others.
- The kind of care you are able to give is conditioned by how you have been treated by parents, teachers and trainers.

If you have been a patient yourself, you might be aware of the powerful expectations that become evident when you need expert help. You make a quite rapid judgement about whether this professional person is in touch with you. This is based more on their ability to see things from your point of view than on their knowledge, status or skill.

We are trained to be objective about disease and its treatment, yet almost everything about the patient journey narrative is just the opposite. It is about the subjective experiences of patients, their parents and their siblings: anxiety, relief, fury, gratitude, terror and grief. Technique and objective knowledge are always necessary, but never sufficient. These days, clinical training makes more of the clinical relationship, but there is still little awareness of the barriers between professional and patient.

The doctor is telling you something about your child who is seriously ill. Your head is spinning. He gives you a leaflet and says that it's all explained there. You wonder if you are going to faint, his voice seems far away. He does not seem to have noticed, so you sit down and look intelligent while feeling quite strange and disconnected.

Here, 'information' means something quite different to the giver and to the receiver, who cannot take it in. A doctor who does not notice that is out of touch.

USING YOUR IMAGINATION: UNDERSTANDING AND BEING UNDERSTOOD

The key to getting in touch as a clinician is to use your imagination and to be observant – about yourself as well as others. What might it be like to be that patient or parent? What do you see in the faces and movements of the people you are talking to? What is your emotional reaction to this particular patient's story?

One junior doctor I worked with in a discussion group was very shocked by her own violent feelings in the presence of a mother who was being cruel to her child. We don't have to accept everything that patients do, but we must be aware of our own reactions. Young clinicians often think they are meant to be kind even to people who abuse them. Some people are just too rude and you have to find a way of saying no.

There is a common theme of gratitude in the parents' narratives when staff make them feel understood, when they don't look away or brusquely send them off to another specialist somewhere else, with no clear idea of when or where the appointment will be. Even polite and obedient patients can feel disorientated, guilty or angry when they don't know what is going on. Just as in giving directions to people who are lost, you cannot assume that patients have the same map in their heads as you have. Making yourself available – for example, via email – to clarify queries or explain results can make a huge difference to families who are in the midst of a stressful time. This is not about being nice, it's about being aware of the bottomless anxiety that 'not knowing' causes.

Mind Your Language

When you want to explain something, you have to mind your language. 'Cerebral palsy', for example, may have quite a specific meaning to *you* because you know your anatomy, physiology and pathology, but very little to a child or parent. If they do happen to have a relative with cerebral palsy or have seen someone with it on television, they may still have a very different image in their mind to the one that you are trying to give them. You can also talk about risk but (unless they are gamblers) it's just numbers to most people. The words you use, such as 'probably' or 'might', can be seriously misinterpreted.[5]

Just like a parent or teacher, it is part of our task to notice if what we are saying is making sense. If you think you are not getting through, the best thing to do is to say something like, 'Maybe I have not explained this clearly enough', or, 'Perhaps this is too difficult to take in at the moment', then stop talking and wait a few moments.

The most difficult thing to impart is a diagnosis of a long-term or fatal disease. I think it is wrong for beginners to have to break bad news, yet many are left to do so.[6] Trainees should first observe their seniors doing it,[7] to see that it is not about telling people you know how they feel (you almost certainly don't). It's about being able to find genuine, normal words to show your respect for their suffering. All you might be able to say is, 'I am so sorry'. You might feel like crying, which is not a terrible thing to do provided you can carry on working. But it is not good practice to switch off just when you need to be paying attention. One mother's narrative recorded her fury with a doctor: 'She asked a few questions and told us he [her son] was delayed without even looking at him'.

> We can learn to tap into and improve reflective skills during training. Though roleplay[8] helps, real clinical settings are the best places to learn, some of which can then be reviewed in case discussions.[9]

WORKING WITH THE SYSTEM AROUND THE PATIENT

In the patient narratives, we often hear about a 'breakdown in communication'. It seems so obvious that if there are people working with your patient (say, in another clinic), then they need to be told about what you have been doing. So why does this link-up so often not happen? First, it may not be clear who is responsible for making that connection, but secondly, there may be a failure of imagination. The boundaries of any case extend beyond the walls of your department. Unless you are conscious of the health and related systems around this patient, you can easily forget about the other people upon whom the family also depends; people they assume you are in communication with. Then the patient goes to another clinic and wonders why they have hardly any information about his or her case:

> No 21st century health system should require parents and children to go from place to place or even worse to go to multiple appointments to tell the same story.[10]

In effect, this leaves the patient or parent in charge of coordinating their own care; a dereliction of our professional duty. Just as in the care of children, there is more security for patients if helping professionals keep in touch with each other. The more complex or disturbing the case, the less likely this is to happen.

Chronic Disease

Most of the patient narratives are about children with disabilities or other long-term conditions. Nothing better illustrates the need for integrated and stable health services in which different organisations keep in contact with one another. In general, disability and chronic disease can turn family life upside down,[11] with the parents having to fit in frequent clinic appointments while trying to run a family with other children who also need looking after. It's not unusual to hear of parents who have split up under the strain.[12] Although all chronic diseases have a significant impact on family life, when the brain is involved, there is likely to be still more distress. In children with epilepsy, for example, rates of emotional and behavioural problems are four-times greater than in the general community.[13] Many more children with chronic and complex disorders could benefit from mental health services that are integrated with medical ones,[14–16] but this sensible idea is frequently forgotten.[17]

Parents make heroic efforts to keep the siblings[18] of their sick child in focus (and the siblings themselves may be heroically patient), but it is a herculean task. Brothers and sisters of any age will feel excluded by the necessary attention lavished on the patient. They might also feel guilty about their own good health and by the fact that they can do so little to heal their ill sibling. Most families in this situation do not get the chance to explore these emotions, and because they are so busy, some may not even think that such an opportunity is necessary.

- Patient narratives show how a lack of authority and imagination within teams, or mistrust between them, undermines integrated care.
- However expert patients and parents become,[19,20] they cannot possibly lead the professional network.
- In every case in which there are several agencies involved, it must be clear to everyone who is the care coordinator.

HOSPITALS

Being in hospital is disturbing for anyone. Everything is unfamiliar; you are expecting some treatment that may be painful and are often utterly dependent on others, like a tiny baby. Just imagine, then, how much more unsettling this is for a child patient.[21] More than anything else, a child in hospital is helped by the presence of one or both of his or her parents, but they themselves will feel insecure because they are not at home and have very little authority to organise anything without asking, even begging for it. Very young children often want to bring their special toy or blanket – 'transitional object'[22] – with them, which is a comfort. Hospital staff need to understand children's anxieties. Our resistance to doing so comes from not wanting to be reminded of how frightening and confusing childhood can be. Cheerful reassurance, such as making jokes, may be tempting, but is unlikely to have any useful effect for more than a moment. Getting paediatricians and children's nurses to allow parents to visit their children in hospital at times that suited them, and then to stay the night with them if they wanted, was an enormous struggle that lasted from the 1950s until the 1980s.[23]

CONCLUSION

Making an accurate judgement about another person's state of mind has nothing to do with sympathetically feeling sorry for them, which can be sentimental and patronising. This chapter is about learning to pay thoughtful attention to your own perceptions and reactions in clinical situations, which then becomes a professional skill.[24] If you can reflect on your emotional capacities as you do your intellectual and technical work, you will be a better clinician. Patients notice that.

REFERENCES

1. Bowlby, J. 1988. *A Secure Base*. London: Routledge.
2. Music, G. 2010. *Nurturing Natures: Attachment and Children's Emotional, Social and Brain Development*. Hove/New York: Psychology Press.
3. Winnicott, D.W. 1960. The theory of the parent–infant relationship. *International Journal of Psycho-Analysis* 41: 585–95.
4. Gerhardt, S. 2015. *Why Love Matters: How Affection Shapes a Baby's Brain* (second edition). London: Routledge.
5. Cohn, L.D., Schydlower, M., Foley, J., Copeland, R.L. 1995. Adolescents' misinterpretation of health risk probability expressions. *Pediatrics* 95(5): 713–6.
6. Orlander, J.D., Fincke, B.G., Hermanns, D., Johnson, G.A. 2002. Medical residents' first clearly remembered experiences of giving bad news. *Journal of General Internal Medicine* 17: 825–31.

7. Conn, R., Berry, P.A. 2010. The decision to engage in end-of-life discussions: A structured approach for doctors in training. *Clinical Medicine* 10(5): 468–71.

8. Greenberg, L., Ochenslager, D., O'Donnell, R., Mastruserio, J., Cohen, G. 1999. Communicating bad news: A pediatric department's evaluation of a simulated intervention. *Pediatrics* 103(6): 1210–7.

9. Shoenberg, P. and Yakely, J. 2014. *Learning about Emotions in Illness*. London: Routledge.

10. Prof. Ian Kennedy speaking at the launch of his review: Getting it right for children and young people. Overcoming cultural barriers in the NHS so as to meet their needs. September 2010, London: COI. (Cited in *BMJ*2010; 341: c5129.)

11. 2005. Chronic childhood illness. *Clinical Child Psychology and Psychiatry* (special issue) 10(1) http://ccp.sagepub.com/content/vol10/issue1/.

12. Berge, J., Patterson, J., Rueter, M. 2006. Marital satisfaction and mental health of couples with children with chronic health conditions. *Families, Systems, & Health* 24(3): 267–85.

13. Davies, S., Heyman, I., Goodman, R. 2003. A population survey of mental health problems in children with epilepsy. *Developmental Medicine and Child Neurology* 45(5): 292–5.

14. Ellenwood, A. and Jenkins, J. 2007. Unbalancing the effects of chronic illness: Non-traditional family therapy assessment and intervention approach. *The American Journal of Family Therapy* 35(3): 265–77.

15. Johnstone, R.J. and Morton, M.J.S. 2009. Specialist mental healthcare for children with epilepsy: Child and adolescent mental health service liaison with neuroscience. *Psychiatric Bulletin* 33: 384–6.

16. Kraemer, S. 2010. Liaison and co-operation between paediatrics and mental health. *Paediatrics and Child Health* 20(8): 382–7.

17. Kraemer, S. 2016. The view from the bridge; Bringing a third position to child health. In S. Campbell, R. Catchpole and D. Morley (eds.). *Child & Adolescent Mental Health: New Insights to Practice*. London: Palgrave Macmillan.

18. Barlow, J. and Ellard, D. 2005. The psychosocial well-being of children with chronic disease, their parents and siblings: An overview of the research evidence base. *Child: Care, Health & Development* 32(1): 19–31.

19. Tuffrey, C. and Finlay, F. 2002. Use of the internet by parents of paediatric outpatients. *Archives of Disease in Childhood* 87: 534–6.

20. Twomey, C. and Busk, M. 2011. Learning from adult services: Expert patients to expert parents. *BMJ Supportive & Palliative Care* 1: 200–1.

21. Kirkby, R. and Whelan, T. 1996. The effects of hospitalisation and medical procedures on children and their families. *Journal of Family Studies* 2: 65–77.

22. Winnicott, D.W. 1953. Transitional objects and transitional phenomena – A study of the first not-me possession. *International Journal of Psycho-Analysis* 34: 89–97.

23. Brandon, S., Lindsey, M., Lovell-Davis, J., Kraemer, S. 2009. 'What is wrong with emotional upset?' – 50 years on from the Platt Report. *Archives of Disease in Childhood* 94: 173–7.

24. Ballatt, J. and Campling, P. 2011. *Intelligent Kindness: Reforming the Culture of Healthcare*. London: RCPsych Publications.

6

Reflections of a Parent

Carol Nahra

When my son Dillon was about to turn 1 – a birthday that we knew would likely be the only one he would have – I started a blog. This was in the days just before social media took off, and for a year I had been pretty isolated, only occasionally communicating via email and telephone. I began detailing our lives in hospital, where Dillon suffered from a debilitating brain condition, to friends and family, and a community which grew by the day. My blog readers from outside our relentlessly shrunken world all wanted to understand what our daily lives were like.

But what I didn't anticipate was how useful my blog would prove for those who we saw regularly. The nurses looking after Dillon began reading it, and felt they had a much better understanding of Dillon's condition, as well as the daily difficulties we faced. The blog gave context to our lives. Whilst Dillon died only 2 months after his first birthday, the blog remains as a vivid snapshot of his final weeks with us.

This book, with its raw, first-person accounts of families living in a difficult medical universe, provides similar snapshots. Reading them transports me straight back into the turbulent days of Dillon's life. Whilst each of these stories is so different, cumulatively they quickly cluster around themes, all of which resonate with my own experience. Some themes, like disjointed services, remain a problem that is unlikely to be resolved soon. But for me, one of the most pervasive themes is also one of the easiest to address: communication.

As an American living in London, when Dillon was born I felt like a true foreigner, despite having lived here for more than a decade. I couldn't understand the language of the hospital, and didn't even understand what a consultant was, or a 'sister'. I could have benefitted from a simple hospital orientation explaining the hierarchy, the shift structure and the bureaucracy. As I write in the chapter on Dillon, what would have been of most use to us as a family would have been a key worker, some sort of saviour who understood everything and could help us through on a daily basis – wishful thinking, I know.

Without the buffer of a key worker, every interaction with professionals for the family is potentially difficult and fraught. In the amplified, dissonant world of a family who is lurching from bad news to bad news, every word matters. Nearly a decade later, it is both the kindest and the harshest interactions that I remember. The brusque moments where an ill-chosen phrase felt like a blow, and also the warming moments, of which there were many, where a nurse or a consultant or a play specialist gave us compassion and time.

No individual communication impacted the fact that we had a very ill baby. But all of them contributed, for bad and for good, to how we coped as a family and how we look back on this period in our lives. So the best advice I can give is to be kind and to explain everything carefully, considerately and patiently. Repeat. Above all, don't forget the context – or the compassion.